HARRIET HAY

Monitoring the Critically Ill Patient

Monitoring the Critically Ill Patient

EDITED BY

Philip Jevon
RGN, BSc (Hon), PGCE, ENB 124
Resuscitation Training Officer
Manor Hospital
Walsall
UK

AND

Beverley Ewens
RN, BSc (Hon), PGCE, ENB 100
Nurse Consultant
Critical Care Services
Manor Hospital
Walsall
UK

CONSULTING EDITOR

Jagtar Singh Pooni
BSc (Hons) MRCP (UK) FRCA
Consultant in Anaesthesia and
Intensive Care Medicine
City Hospital
Birmingham
UK

Blackwell
Science

Editorial offices:
Blackwell Science Ltd, 9600 Garsington Road, Oxford OX4 2DQ, UK
  Tel: +44 (0) 1865 776868
Blackwell Publishing Inc., 350 Main Street, Malden, MA 02148-5020, USA
  Tel: +1 781 388 8250
Blackwell Science Asia Pty, 550 Swanston Street, Carlton, Victoria 3053,
Australia
  Tel: +61 (0)3 8359 1011

First published 2002
Reprinted 2003 (twice)

Library of Congress Cataloging-in-Publication Data
Monitoring the critically ill patient/edited by Philip Jevon and
Beverley Ewens.
    p.   ;   cm.
  Includes bibliographical references and index.
  ISBN 0-632-05803-X (alk. paper)
  1. Patient monitoring.   2. Critical care medicine.   I. Jevon, Philp.
II. Ewens, Beverley.
  [DNLM: 1. Intensive Care—methods.   2. Monitoring, Physiologic—
methods.   3. Critical Illness. WX 218 M7444 2002]
RT48.55 .M665 2002
616'.028—dc21

2001043022

ISBN 0-632-05803-X

A catalogue record for this title is available from the British Library

Set in 8 on 12pt Palatino
by SNP Best-set Typesetters Ltd., Hong Kong
Printed and bound in Great Britain using acid-free paper
by MPG Books Ltd, Bodmin, Cornwall

For further information on Blackwell Publishing, visit our website:
www.blackwellpublishing.com

Contents

Foreword

Ian Dyer
RN, Di N, DipMgt, ENB 998, ENB 100, B Tech (Hons), MSc, PhD
Manager Critical Care Units
Walsall Manor Hospital, UK

Until fairly recently most hospital staff perceived 'critical care' as a designated unit where the sickest patients are cared for. However, the well publicised shortage of critical care beds in the UK has led to a reappraisal of the provision of critical care services (DoH, 2000, 2001) and to the realisation that critical care is not a location, but an approach to the way that care is provided.

Although the number of critical care unit beds has increased, and this expansion is likely to continue, there is a recognition that critical care can, and should be, if necessary, provided to patients outside designated units. This approach has been described as providing 'critical care without walls' – the provision of critical care interventions when and where the patient needs them. Monitoring is a key component of this care. It allows the early detection of potential problems so that patients can either be admitted to critical care units before problems become severe or so that treatment can be initiated and deterioration (which could lead to the need for admission to a critical care unit) avoided.

The consequence of this changing approach is that all staff involved in the care of acutely ill patients should understand the principles of monitoring. In one sense this is nothing new. The condition of a patient has always been monitored and anyone who has taken a pulse or measured urine output has been engaged in monitoring. Clinical observational skills are as important now as they ever were, but they are no longer sufficient. To these clinical skills carers must add an understanding of the technological aspects of monitoring; how and when the various techniques are used; how to troubleshoot problems; how to interpret the information provided and how to integrate clinical and technical information to better understand the condition of patients under their care.

The authors have many years of experience in the monitoring of critically ill patients both within and outside of critical care units. This book distils their experience and provides staff involved in acute care with the knowledge of and the skills in monitoring which they need to provide safe and high quality care. It takes a systematic approach which describes the clinical and technical aspects of monitoring of the lungs; heart; neurological system; kidneys; gut and nutritional status; liver; endocrine system and temperature. Chapters begin by describing the clinical and observation skills which are the basis of high quality care and uses these to introduce the more technical aspects of monitoring. For each physiological system the book provides descriptions of relevant clinical conditions and illustrates these with scenarios which will allow readers to test their developing knowledge.

Effective application of the techniques described will improve patient care in ward areas and will also allow the detection of problems which require admission to critical care units. To support this the book concludes with chapters on the transport of critically ill patients and record keeping which will make the transfer of patients to these units as safe as possible.

The information provided is relevant to all health care professionals involved in acute care, for:

- student nurses it provides a concise and comprehensive introduction to monitoring which will help them to develop the clinical acumen required to provide safe and high quality care
- nurses working on acute wards it summarises and adds to the clinical knowledge which they will already possess and describes the use of monitoring equipment which is increasingly becoming part of their everyday practice
- nurses and junior doctors working in high dependency and critical care units it provides a grounding in the technical aspects of

monitoring which they can build on as they develop their skills and experience
- allied health professionals who are involved in the care of acutely ill patients, it explains the technical aspects of patient care which they will meet in their daily work.

This book is not the final word in monitoring. No single book ever could be, and monitoring techniques will continue to develop, but it is an ideal introduction to the subject and provides a basis for more advanced learning.

REFERENCES

DoH (2000) *Comprehensive Critical Care. A Review of Adult Critical Care Services.* Department of Health, London.
DoH (2001) *The Nursing Contribution to the Provision of Comprehensive Critical Care for Adults.* Department of Health, London.

Preface

Welcome to the first edition of *Monitoring the Critically Ill Patient*. Generally, patients are now older, sicker, more dependent and more likely to have co-existing morbidity. In addition the management of critically ill patients is becoming commonplace outside the intensive care environment.

Nurses, whether they are working in intensive care units or on generally wards, must have the necessary knowledge and expertise to accurately and safely monitor critically ill patients. The early detection of problems, together with appropriate management, is paramount.

This book provides the reader with a systematic and comprehensive approach to the monitoring of a critically ill patient. We hope that nurses will find it an invaluable resource.

Philip Jevon and Beverley Ewens
December 2001

Acknowledgements

The authors are grateful to:

- Jagtar Singh Pooni, consultant in Anaesthesia and Intensive Care Medicine at City Hospital in Birmingham, for his help with writing Chapters 2 and 12 and for kindly agreeing to be consultant editor for the book;
- John Hamilton and his staff at the Medical Photography Department at the Manor Hospital in Walsall for their assistance with photographs;
- Laerdal Medical for providing the ECG traces;
- Tim Simmons, formally Senior Charge Nurse on ITU at the Manor Hospital in Walsall for his help with Chapter 9;
- Dee Cope, Nurse Specialist on Neuro ITU at University Hospital, Birmingham, for her help with Chapter 4;
- *Nursing Times* for granting us permission to reproduce material from an article we wrote for them;
- Cambridge University Press, Butterworth-Heinemann, Churchill Livingstone, Baillière Tindall, routledge and Oxford University Press for kindly granting us permission to reproduce material from their publications.

Monitoring Respiratory Function

1

INTRODUCTION

The symptoms of respiratory disease may be insignificant or extremely distressing for the patient; either may indicate a serious or life threatening disease (Johnson, 1987). Respiratory function requires careful and close monitoring to ensure the most appropriate treatment is administered and any response to it accurately evaluated. Table 1.1 shows the basic definitions of respiratory terminology and Table 1.2 some of the most common causes of dyspnoea (breathing difficulty).

In particular it is important to be able to recognise when the patient's respiratory status is compromised. The familiar *look*, *listen* and *feel* approach can be used to evaluate the efficacy of breathing, work of breathing and adequacy of ventilation. The patient's general appearance, history and presenting symptoms together with the characteristics of the dyspnoea are also important. Peak flow measurements, pulse oximetry and blood gas analysis are also helpful in monitoring respiratory function.

The aim of this chapter is to understand the principles of monitoring respiratory function.

LEARNING OBJECTIVES

At the end of the chapter the reader will be able to:

❏ describe how to assess the *efficacy of breathing, work of breathing* and *adequacy of ventilation*;

❏ discuss the importance of a *comprehensive assessment* of the patient;

Table 1.1 Definitions of respiratory terminology

Dyspnoea	difficulty in breathing
Orthopnoea	dyspnoea necessitating an upright, sitting position for its relief
Tachypnoea	abnormally rapid rate of breathing (>20 per minute) (Torrance & Elley 1997)
Bradypnoea	abnormally slow rate of breathing (<12 per minute) (Torrance & Elley 1997)
Hypoxia	inadequate oxygen at cellular level
Hypoxaemia	low oxygen levels in the blood
Anoxia	lack of oxygen, local or systemic

Table 1.2 Causes of dyspnoea (not exhaustive)

Respiratory	e.g. asthma, chronic obstructive pulmonary disease (COPD), pneumonia, tuberculosis, pleural effusion, pneumothorax, carcinoma of the lung, pulmonary embolism; mechanical, e.g. fractured ribs – flail segment
Cardiac	e.g. left ventricular failure & pulmonary oedema, congestive cardiac failure
CNS	e.g. head injury, raised intracranial pressure, drugs, e.g. opiates; aggravating factors e.g. exercise, cold air, smoking, coughing
Neuromuscular	e.g. Guillain–Barre syndrome, myasthenia gravis, muscular dystrophies
Diabetes	hyperventilation in ketoacidosis
Pregnancy	
Obesity	
Anaemia	

Adapted from Jevon & Ewews 2001

❏ outline important *associated features of dyspnoea*;
❏ describe how to undertake *peak expiratory flow rate measurements*;
❏ discuss the principles of *pulse oximetry*;
❏ discuss the principles of *arterial blood gas analysis*;
❏ discuss the monitoring priorities of a *ventilated patient*;
❏ outline the monitoring priorities of a *patient with a chest drain*.

ASSESSMENT OF THE EFFICACY OF BREATHING, WORK OF BREATHING AND ADEQUACY OF VENTILATION

Efficacy of breathing

The efficacy of breathing can be assessed by the following.

- *Air entry*: look, listen and feel for signs of breathing. If able, auscultate the chest to determine the amount of air being inspired/expired in the apices and bases. A silent chest is an ominous sign.
- *Chest movement*: is chest movement equal, bilateral and symmetrical? The depth of inspiration should be noted.
- *Pulse oximetry*: continuous oxygen saturation monitoring.
- *Arterial blood gas analysis*: the definitive method to assess the effectiveness of ventilation.

Work of breathing

Healthy spontaneous breathing is quiet and accomplished with minimal effort (Jevon & Ewens 2001). Signs of increased work of breathing include a rise in *respiratory rate*, *noisy respirations* and *use of accessory muscles*.

Respiratory rate

The normal respiratory rate in adults is approximately 12 breaths per minute; tachypnoea is usually one of the first indications of respiratory distress (bradypnoea may be an ominous sign and possible causes include drugs, e.g. opiates, fatigue, hypothermia and CNS depression). The following disturbed breathing patterns are also significant:

- *Kussmaul's breathing (air hunger)*: deep rapid respirations due to stimulation of the respiratory centre by metabolic acidosis, e.g. in ketoacidosis or chronic renal failure;
- *Cheyne-Stokes breathing pattern*: periods of apnoea alternating with periods of hyperpnoea; causes include left ventricular failure and cerebral injury; usually seen in the end stages of life;
- *Hyperventilation*: often associated with anxiety states.

Noisy respirations
The following symptoms are also indicative of breathing difficulty.

- *Stridor*: 'croaking' respiration which is louder during inspiration; caused by laryngeal or tracheal obstruction, e.g. foreign body, laryngeal oedema or laryngeal tumour.
- *Wheeze* – noisy musical sound caused by turbulent flow of air through narrowed bronchi and bronchioles, more pronounced on expiration; causes include asthma and chronic obstructive pulmonary disease (COPD).
- *'Rattly' chest*: e.g. chest infection, pulmonary oedema and sputum retention.
- *Gurgling*: caused by fluid in the upper airway.
- *Snoring*: snoring sounds may be associated with the tongue blocking the airway in an unconscious patient.

Jevon & Ewens 2001

Accessory muscle use
The use of accessory muscles, e.g. neck and abdominal muscles is a further indication of breathing difficulty.

Adequacy of ventilation
The assessment of heart rate, skin colour and the patient's mental status can help provide an indication of the adequacy of ventilation. Hypoxaemia can affect the following.

- *Heart rate*: initially tachycardia (a non-specific sign), but severe hypoxia can cause bradycardia;
- *Skin colour*: initially pallor, hypoxia causes catecholamine release and vasoconstriction; central cyanosis is a late and often preterminal sign of hypoxia (if the patient is anaemic, severe hypoxaemia may not cause cyanosis).*
- *Mental status*: agitation (may be an early sign), drowsiness, confusion and impaired consciousness.

(Jevon & Ewens 2001)

*NB if the patient has chronic obstructive pulmonary disorder (COPD) or congenital heart disease, cyanosis may be 'constant'.

COMPREHENSIVE ASSESSMENT OF THE PATIENT

The following matters should all be investigated and taken into account to arrive at a comprehensive assessment of the patient's condition.

Severity

It is important to establish what is normal for the patient and the effect of the breathlessness on the patient (Jevon & Ewens 2001): e.g. can the patient talk with ease? How far can the patient walk without having to stop? Can the patient climb the stairs? Is the patient orthopnoeic? If so how many pillows does the patient sleep with? Does breathlessness affect the patient's daily activities or job? Does the patient require oxygen at home? (Jevon & Ewens 2001)

Timing

Severe asthma and left ventricular failure is more common at night. Occupation related asthma is worse when the patient is at work and improves when the patient is at home (Jevon & Ewens 2001). Bronchitis is more common in the winter months.

Finger clubbing

Finger clubbing can indicate pulmonary or cardiovascular disease; clinical features often include loss of nailbed angle, an increased curvature of the nail and swelling of the terminal part of the digit (Johnson 1987).

Shape of the chest
The normal chest is bilaterally symmetrical, though it can be distorted by disease of the ribs or spinal vertebrae as well as by underlying lung disease. In kyphosis (forward bending) or scoliosis (lateral bending) of the vertebral column, lung movement can be severely restricted. A barrel chest is sometimes associated with chronic bronchitis and emphysema (Jevon & Ewens 2001).

Chest percussion
Hyper-resonance to percussion is caused by an increase in air in the chest, e.g. emphysema, pneumothorax. Dullness to percussion can be caused by thickening of the chest wall, lung consolidation or pleural effusion.

Auscultation of the chest
Diminished breath sounds can be caused by poor ventilation, e.g. airway obstruction, respiratory depression or by increased separation of the stethoscope from the bronchial tree, e.g. obesity, pleural effusion, pneumothorax, bronchial tumour. Fine crackles (crepitations) may be heard, e.g. pulmonary oedema; a pleural rub or inflammation of the pleura.

Medications
Medications the patient is currently taking may be significant. For instance, beta blockers can exacerbate asthma and left ventricular failure.

Halitosis
This may indicate poor oral hygiene or could be a sign of an infection of the upper respiratory tract.

Patient's position and emotional state

Does the patient need to sit in a particular position, e.g. supported by a bed-table to facilitate breathing? Is the patient orthopneic? A breathless patient will be anxious.

Past medical history and family medical history

All previous illnesses, operations, hospital admissions and investigations, particularly those that are respiratory related, should be noted. Has the patient been prescribed any respiratory related medication, e.g. inhalers or oxygen? If so the frequency and effectiveness of its use should be noted. Any respiratory disease in the patient's family should be noted.

Occupational and social history

When assessing respiratory disease, both past and present occupations together with any exposure to dust, asbestos, coal or animals could be significant. If the patient smokes, past and present consumption should be noted together with any exposure to infection, e.g. tuberculosis. The type of living accommodation may be significant, e.g. stairs, damp environment, lack of a working lift in a block of flats.

Patient's age

Certain respiratory diseases are more likely to occur at particular times of life: <30 years – asthma, pneumothorax, cystic fibrosis, congenital heart disease; >50 years – chronic bronchitis, chronic obstructive pulmonary disorder (COPD), carcinoma of the lung, pneumoconiosis, ischaemic heart disease.

Racial background or recent travel

Patients who have recently arrived from the Asian subcontinent may have been exposed to tuberculosis.

Allergies

Any allergies should be recorded in both the patient's medical and nursing notes and on the prescription administration chart.

ASSOCIATED SYMPTOMS OF DYSPNOEA

Chest pain

Respiratory related chest pain or pleuritic pain is usually sharp in nature and aggravated by deep breathing or coughing. It is often localised to one particular area (Jevon & Ewens 2001).

Cough

A cough is a common respiratory symptom. It occurs when deep inspiration is followed by an explosive expiration. A cough that is worse at night is suggestive of asthma or heart failure, while a cough that is worse after eating is suggestive of oesophageal reflux. The timing and duration of the cough is important:

- *sudden cough*: may be due to a foreign body;
- *recent cough*: may be due to a chest infection;
- *chronic cough associated with a wheeze*: may be due to asthma;
- *irritating chronic dry cough*: may be due to oesophageal reflux;
- *chronic cough with production of large volumes of purulent sputum*: may be due to bronchiectasis;
- *change in the character of a chronic cough*: may be due to a serious underlying pathology, e.g. carcinoma of the lung.

Jevon & Ewens 2001

Sputum

Sputum is a key clinical feature of respiratory disease and can provide valuable information for the assessment of a breathless patient, including evaluation of care (Law 2000). If sputum is produced, its colour and consistency should be noted:

- *white mucoid sputum*: seen in asthma and chronic bronchitis;
- *purulent green or yellow sputum*: may indicate respiratory infection;
- *blood present*: may indicate carcinoma of the lung, pulmonary embolism (Brewis 1996);
- *frothy white or pink sputum*: seen in pulmonary oedema;

- *thick, viscid sputum*: feature of severe or life-threatening asthma (Rees & Price 1999);
- *thin, watery sputum*: associated with acute pulmonary oedema (Middleton & Middleton 1998);
- *foul smelling sputum*: indication of respiratory tract infection;
- *black specks*: common causes include smoke inhalation and coal dust.

The patient's history is important when determining the significance of sputum production at a particular time of day, e.g. chronic expectoration in the morning over a number of years may be suggestive of smoking-induced bronchitis while variable morning or nocturnal expectoration may be suggestive of asthma (Law 2000).

Important coexisting clinical features

A number of important coexisting clinical features may be associated with respiratory problems, including:

- *fever*: respiratory infection;
- *poor appetite and weight loss*: carcinoma of the lung, chronic infection;
- *swollen and painful calf*: deep vein thrombosis and pulmonary embolism;
- *ankle swelling*: congestive cardiac failure, deep vein thrombosis;
- *palpitations*: cardiac arrhythmias.

Jevon & Ewens 2001

MEASUREMENT OF PEAK EXPIRATORY FLOW RATE

Peak expiratory flow rate (PEFR) or peak flow is the maximum flow rate attained on forced expiration from a position of full inspiration. It is a simple test to ascertain the severity of a patient's asthma and can provide the practitioner with a guide to the level of resistance within the bronchioles. This resistance can be caused by inflammation and/or bronchospasm. Peak flow is not a measure of fitness or the strength of the patient's chest muscles.

Indications

Recordings should be undertaken four times a day, both before and after the administration of bronchodilators (Ross-Plummer 2000). The results are crucial to the patient's treatment and are an indicator to how well the patient's asthma is responding to treatment.

Normal range for peak expiratory flow rate measurements

The normal range for peak flow recordings is influenced by age, sex and height (Nunn & Gregg 1989). Peak flow readings are usually higher in men than women and the best peak flow usually occurs between the ages of 30–40 (Partridge 1997). In addition it varies throughout the day; it is often higher in the evenings than in the mornings. It is therefore important to record peak flows at both these times.

Procedure

(1) Explain the procedure to the patient.
(2) Assemble the necessary equipment – mini-Wright flow meter, clean mouth piece, observation chart. Ensure the flow meter is set at zero.
(3) If possible stand the patient up.
(4) Ask the patient to take a deep breath in and place the peak flow meter in the mouth, holding it horizontally and closing the lips.
(5) Ask the patient to breathe out as hard and as fast as possible.
(6) Note the recording on the flow meter and then return it to zero.
(7) Ask the patient to repeat the procedure twice.
(8) Record the best of the three recordings.

Adapted from Jevon *et al*. 2000

PRINCIPLES OF PULSE OXIMETRY

Pulse oximetry is probably the greatest advance in patient monitoring since the invention of the ECG. It is a simple, non-invasive method of continuous monitoring of oxygenation, an important physiological variable that is poorly detected by clinical means (Hanning & Alexander-Williams 1995).

Although pulse oximetry is useful for detecting hypoxaemia (Hutton & Clutton-Brock 1993), as with any aspect of technology, it is merely an aid to observation and total patient care, not a substitute (Woodrow 1999). Nevertheless, it is an invaluable monitoring tool in a variety of clinical settings, as long as its uses and limitations are fully understood (Jevon & Ewens 2000).

Role of pulse oximetry

Hypoxaemia is common in all aspects of medical practice and is a major cause of organ dysfunction and death (Hanning & Alexander-Williams 1995). Unfortunately the visual detection of cyanosis, the traditional sign of hypoxaemia, is subject to considerable observer bias.

When the oxygen saturation falls to 89%, cyanosis is detected by experienced practitioners in only 95% of patients. Several studies have shown that even under ideal conditions skilled practitioners are unable to detect hypoxaemia until the oxygen saturation is <80% (Comroe & Botelho 1947). In addition, delayed manifestations of hypoxaemia including restlessness, confusion, agitation, cyanosis and tachycardia may be missed or wrongly interpreted (Technology Subcommittee of the Working Group on Critical Care 1992).

Pulse oximetry will immediately alert the practitioner to a fall in arterial oxygen saturations and the development of hypoxaemia. In general terms an oxygen saturation of less than 90% is of concern. NB the absence of cyanosis does not exclude severe hypoxaemia; it will not be present if the haemoglobin concentration is low or if there is poor perfusion of the capillaries.

The mechanics of pulse oximetry

The pulse oximeter (Fig. 1.1) works on the principle of Beer's Law: the concentration of an unknown solute dissolved in a solvent can be determined by light absorption (Lynne *et al.* 1990). Anything which pulses and absorbs red and infrared light between the light detector and the light source must be arterial blood (Lowton 1999).

The amount of light absorption when applied to a digit varies between oxygen-rich and oxygen-poor haemoglobin; haemoglobin oxygen saturation can then be estimated by measuring the difference of absorption between full (systole) and empty (diastole) capillaries (Woodrow 1999). The difference of light absorption is calculated over a number of pulses (Harrahill 1991).

The pulse oximeter probe consists of two light-emitting diodes (one red and one infrared) on one side of the probe.

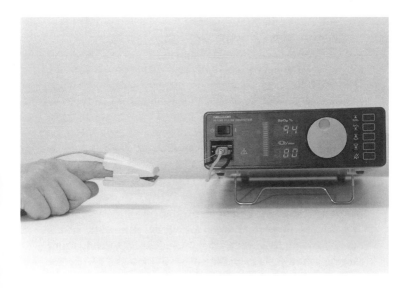

Fig. 1.1 Pulse oximeter

These transmit red and infrared light through body tissue, usually a finger tip or ear lobe, to a photodetector on the other side of the probe. A micropressor processes or filters the signals received and provides a digital display of oxygen saturation symbolised by SpO_2 (Jenson *et al*. 1998).

Uses of pulse oximetry

Pulse oximetry is indicated in any clinical situation where hypoxaemia may occur (Hanning & Alexander-Williams 1995). It is used in a variety of clinical settings including:

- theatres;
- intensive care units;
- general wards;
- neonatal units;
- patient transfer;
- sleep studies;
- primary care.

Advantages of pulse oximetry

Pulse oximetry is an inexpensive non-invasive method of continuous measurement of arterial oxygen saturation which facilitates the early detection of hypoxaemia. It also provides information about the heart rate (Jevon & Ewens 2000).

Although analysis of arterial blood gases has been the gold standard for measuring arterial oxygen saturation, it is invasive, time-consuming, costly, involves repeated arterial blood sampling and only provides intermittent information (Jenson *et al*. 1998).

Normal values for oxygen saturation

The normal range for oxygen saturation measurements is 95–100% (Hinds & Watson 1996), though lower measurements may be 'normal' in some patients. A sustained trend of falling oxygen saturation levels is clinically important even if the precision of individual readings is poor (Hutton & Clutton-

Brock 1993), though evaluation of other parameters is also important.

Procedure for pulse oximetry
The following preliminary points should be observed:

- ensure the probe is clean;
- wash and dry hands;
- explain the procedure to the patient.

Select an appropriate site with an adequate pulsating vascular bed. Sites include finger (most popular), ear lobe (less accurate, Jenson *et al*. 1998); toes can be used instead of fingers, but poor perfusion is more common (Hanning & Alexander-Williams 1995). Avoid application of the probe distal to blood pressure cuffs or arterial/venous lines. If the finger is used, remove any nail polish (obtain patient's consent first). The probe should be secured, but without the use of restrictive tape. The following precautions must be taken during the procedure:

- ensure that the trace is reliable, i.e. oxygen saturation measurements are accurate (Fig. 1.2);
- ensure the alarms on the pulse oximeter are set within locally agreed limits and according to the patient's condition;
- regularly monitor the probe site for complications, e.g. burns and joint stiffness and regularly vary the site;
- regularly monitor the patient's vital signs;
- document the readings and inform medical staff as appropriate.

Adapted from Jevon & Ewens 2000

Interpreting plethysmographic waveforms
The quality of the pulse and circulation at the point where SpO_2 is being measured is reflected in the plethysmographic waveform (Fig. 1.2); the strength of the pulse is proportional to the amplitude of the waveform (Place 2000).

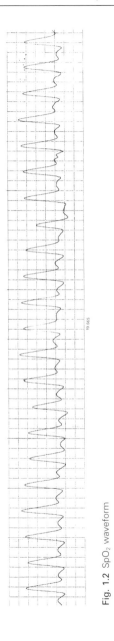

Fig. 1.2 SpO$_2$ waveform

Causes of inaccuracy

Inaccurate readings can be caused by any of the factors listed below.

- *Carbon monoxide poisoning*: false high readings (Stoneham *et al.* 1994).
- *Methaemglobinaemia* (changes in the structure of iron in haemoglobin): can inhibit oxygen release from the haemoglobin resulting in tissue hypoxia and unreliable oxygen saturation measurements (Reynolds *et al.* 1993). Can be caused by lignocaine, nitrates and metoclopramide (Smith & Olson 1989), and local anaesthetics (Coleman & Coleman 1996).
- *Poor vascular perfusion*: pulse oximeter requires pulsatile blood flow to evaluate oxygen saturation.
- *Venous pulsation*: e.g. tight securing of probe (Mackreth 1990), right sided heart failure, inflating blood pressure cuff distal to the probe, resulting in a false low reading.
- *Poor vascular perfusion*: e.g. in hypovolaemia, hypotension, septicaemia, hypothermia, cardiogenic shock or peripheral vascular disease, resulting in a false low reading.
- *Cardiac arrhythmias* such as atrial fibrillation can cause inadequate and irregular perfusion, resulting in a false low reading.
- *Factors that affect light absorption*: e.g. some types of bilirubin (Dobson 1993); dark skin, dried blood and black or blue nail polish (Wahr & Tremper 1996), brown-red nail polish (Cote *et al.* 1988) and intravenous dyes, e.g. methylene blue.
- *Bright external light*, particularly fluorescent lighting (Ralston *et al.* 1991) can give a false high reading.
- *Anaemia* (Severinghaus & Koh 1990 and Weston Smith *et al.* 1989).
- *Patient on supplementary oxygen* can mean that hypoxaemia will not be detected early (Hutton & Clutton-Brock 1993).
- *Oxygen saturations ≤70%* (Schnapp & Cohen 1990).

- *Patient movement*, e.g. shivering; though modern pulse oximeters can minimise the interference from patient movement.

Limitations

Although pulse oximetry measures oxygen saturation and can detect hypoxaemia, it does not provide an indication to the adequacy of ventilation and carbon dioxide retention.

Davidson and Hosie (1993) reported a case of a postoperative patient who had a normal oxygen saturation (95%), but had abnormally high carbon dioxide levels causing a life-threatening respiratory acidosis. Failure to detect hypoventilation in such a patient is an example of a false sense of security generated by a single physiological variable being within safe limits (Hutton & Clutton-Brock 1993).

Trouble shooting

It is important to ensure a reliable trace at all times. If it is difficult to secure an acceptable trace:
- warm and rub the skin to improve circulation;
- try a different probe site, e.g. ear lobe;
- try a different probe/different pulse oximeter.

Complications

Pulse oximetry is very safe; complications are uncommon and are rarely serious if they do occur (Richardson & Hale 1995). Nevertheless complications have been reported.

- *Ischaemic pressure necrosis* (Berge *et al.* 1988): in the reported case the patient was septic, hypotensive and had pre-existing arterial disease. In addition an arterial line was *in situ* in the radial artery which may have further compromised the distal circulation.
- *Perioperative corneal abrasions*: resulting from patients rubbing their eyes with the index finger with probe and dressing attached (Brocke-Utne 1992).

- *Blister injuries at the probe site*: caused by a faulty probe cable; intermittent shortening resulting in excess electrical current supply to the light-emitting diode causing overheating.
- *Mechanical injury*: if the patient is unable to flex his finger; in unconscious or semiconscious patients the probe may inhibit voluntary use of the finger, resulting in stiffness. Changing the probe site regularly is therefore advocated (Richardson & Hale 1995). This is potentially a problem for patients on ICUs where prolonged monitoring occurs.

Best practice – pulse oximetry

Remove anything that could impair the translucence of the sensor site.

Position the probe without excessive force, i.e. use of adhesive tape.

Ensure an accurate trace is obtained.

Note any activity associated with a lower and higher SpO_2 reading.

Always rely on clinical judgement rather than an SpO_2 reading in isolation.

Regularly monitor and alternate probe site.

Ensure the digit used is regularly flexed to avoid mechanical injury.

PRINCIPLES OF ARTERIAL BLOOD GAS ANALYSIS

Arterial blood gas (ABG) analysis is one of the most common tests ordered in the critically ill patient. It provides clinicians with valuable information on a patient's respiratory function and acid base balance (Shoulders-Odom 2000) and as such forms an integral component of monitoring the critically ill patient.

Procedure for arterial blood sampling

There are two methods of arterial blood sampling, either from a one off arterial puncture or 'stab' or from an arterial cannula. An arterial 'stab' is usually taken from the radial artery, as it is most accessible. The femoral artery is also sometimes used.

The following procedure for arterial blood sampling is based on recommendations by Driscoll *et al.* (1997).

(1) Ensure the three way tap is closed to air. This is to prevent back-flow of blood and blood spillage.

(2) Remove cap from three way tap, clean the open port with an alcohol swab and connect a sterile 5 ml syringe.

(3) Turn the tap to connect the artery to the syringe and aspirate 5 ml of blood. This will ensure that the sample of blood used for analysis is fresh and does not contain 'flush solution'. The tap is now 'off' to the flush solution.

(4) Turn the tap off to the syringe; remove and discard the syringe.

(5) Replace with a heparinised syringe and turn the tap to connect it to the artery.

(6) Slowly aspirate the required amount of blood (Fig. 1.3) and then turn the tap off to the syringe. It is important to aspirate the blood slowly as this will help to prevent spasm in the vessel (Mallett & Dougherty 2000).

(7) Remove the syringe and re-apply a new sterile cap, ensuring it is securely attached.

(8) Flush the tubing and watch for return of reliable arterial trace on the monitor. Ensure that the infuser cuff is inflated to 300 mmHg (Mallett & Dougherty 2000).

(9) Undertake arterial blood gas (ABG) analysis following the manufacturer's recommendations ensuring to include the patient's temperature and any supplementary oxygen being administered (Fig. 1.4).

(10) Document the results and inform medical staff if appropriate.

Indications for ABG analysis

Indications for ABG analysis include:

- respiratory compromise;
- post cardiopulmonary arrest;

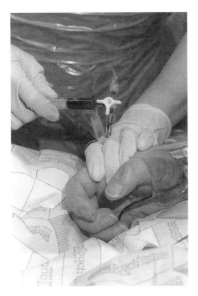

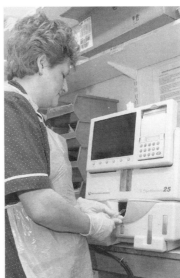

Fig. 1.3 Arterial blood sampling   Fig. 1.4 Blood gas machine

- evaluation of interventions, e.g. changes in ventilation, use of respiratory stimulants, etc.;
- prior to major surgery, to facilitate post operative comparison.

Principles of ABG analysis

Oxygen supply to the tissues is dependent upon how oxygen disassociates itself from the haemoglobin (Hb) molecule to be made available for the tissues. This in turn is dependent upon blood pH, body temperature and PCO_2 of the blood (Hubbard & Mechan 1997). As the blood becomes more acidotic, warmer and with a higher PCO_2, the oxygen dissociation curve shifts to the right and reduces the Hb molecule's affinity for O_2 (Athern et al. 1995). Although less oxygen can be picked up by the lungs, more can be released to the tissues (Valenti et al. 1997). Conversely a shift to the left results in the Hb molecule having a greater affinity to oxygen but less can be released to the tissues. Therefore this may result in poor oxygenation despite an adequate PaO_2.

When a sample of arterial blood is processed by a blood gas analyser it provides not only an invaluable and accurate insight into the patient's respiratory function but also provides a window into their metabolic status.

The levels of blood gases are dependent upon three variables: blood supply, ventilation and diffusion. Therefore if there is a poor blood supply to the alveoli but adequate ventilation insufficient diffusion will lead to a retention of PCO_2, e.g. pulmonary embolus. Conversely if there is a good blood supply to the alveoli but poor ventilation, gaseous exchange will also be compromised, e.g. COPD, pneumonia and asthma. Both of these imbalances will lead to a perfusion ventilation (VQ) mismatch or a 'shunt'. Maximum efficiency in gas exchange between blood and alveoli results when ventilation and perfusion correspond equally (Athern *et al.* 1995).

Blood gas units of measurement are kilopascals (kPa) or millimetres of mercury (mmHg). Both units are currently in use (to convert kPa to mmHg: kPa$\times$7.5 = mmHg and to convert mmHg to kPa: mmHg$\div$7.5 = kPa).

Parameters measured by a blood gas analyser

Arterial blood gas analysis measures several different parameters, as listed below.

- pH: 7.35–7.45 represents the acidity or alkalinity of blood and is a reflection of free H+ ions circulating in the blood.
- PO_2: (10–13.3 kPa) this is the measurement of partial pressure of dissolved oxygen in the blood, usually 2% of O_2 supply (Athern *et al.* 1995). Critically ill patients have increased O_2 demands because of the pathological demands of the body (Shoulders-Odom 2000).
- PCO_2: (4.6–6.0 kPa) measurement of partial pressure of dissolved carbon dioxide in the blood (more soluble than

Table 1.3 Normal ranges for ABG results

pH	7.35–7.45
PO_2	10.0–13.3 kPa
PCO_2	4.6–6.0 kPa
Bicarbonate (HCO_3)	22–26 mmol/l
SaO_2	>95%
Base excess	−2 to +2

© Sheila K. Adam and Sue Osborne 1997. Reproduced by permission of Oxford University Press from Adam & Osborne 1997

oxygen). This is a major source of acid in the body when dissolved in water: $H_2O + CO_2 <> H_2CO_3$ – carbonic acid then dissolves into free H+ ions and bicarbonate H_2CO_3 $HCO_3 + H^+$. Therefore the higher the level of CO_2, the greater the respiratory acidosis.

- HCO_3 (22–26 mmol/l) carries 80% of CO_2 from the tissues to the lungs and is one of the metabolic buffers present in the body – other buffers include Hb, phosphate (PO_4) and plasma proteins (Thibodeau & Patton 1999).
- SaO_2: the percentage of O_2 that has combined with the Hb molecule. O_2 combines with Hb in sufficient amounts to meet needs of the body, whilst at the same time releasing O_2 to meet tissue demands (Shoulders-Odom 2000). The acceptable range is usually 92–99%.
- BE: base excess is an indicator of the amount of buffers available. BE is positive in metabolic alkalosis and negative in metabolic acidosis.
- Electrolytes: most analysers measure electrolytes, e.g. sodium (Na), potassium (K) calcium (Ca) and chloride (Cl) which can be useful for a 'quick check'.

Normal ranges for ABG analysis are shown in Table 1.3.

Systematic analysis of ABG results

Driscoll *et al.* (1997) recommend three steps in analysing ABG results:

- consider the patient's clinical history and physical examination;
- systematically analyse the results;
- integrate the clinical findings with interpretation of the data.

A systematic approach for the analysis of ABG results will now be described.

Step 1
Establish the pH (normal pH 7.35–7.45). Is there is a metabolic imbalance, either acidosis (<7.35) or alkalosis (>7.45)?

Step 2
Examine PCO_2 level (normal 4.6–13.3 kPa). Is it raised or lowered and if so by what degree: mild, moderate or high? This is important when defining the origin of the acidosis/alkalosis and if there are compensatory mechanisms in play.

Step 3
Examine PO_2 level (normal 10.0–13.3 kPa). Is hypoxaemia present? PO_2 has no relevance to acid base balance, only to respiratory function.

Step 4
Examine the bicarbonate level (normal 22–26 mmol/l). Bicarbonate provides an indication to the level of this alkaline buffer in the body, i.e. an indicator of the metabolic state of the patient and classification of the imbalance present.

Step 5
Examine the base excess or deficit (normal +2 to −2). Base excess provides an indication of the severity of an acidosis or an alkalosis, i.e. how much excess or deficit of alkaline is present. If the reading is positive there is a base excess, if negative a base deficit, i.e. there are not enough base products to buffer excess acid. Base excess is also used in calculating the dose of sodium bicarbonate to be administered; however, this

is now used very infrequently as metabolic alkalosis is very difficult to correct, may precipitate cellular acidosis and produces a shift to the left on the oxygen dissociation curve inhibiting release of oxygen to the tissues (Resuscitation Council UK 2000).

Step 6

Examine the SaO_2 level of arterial oxygenation (normal is >95%). If there is low SaO_2 this can indicate a VQ mismatch or 'shunt', i.e. at the level of alveolar gas exchange there is adequate perfusion and inadequate ventilation or inadequate perfusion and adequate ventilation. Shunting of deoxygenated blood causes a decrease in SaO_2 and reduced O_2 to the tissues. For instance pulmonary embolus results in inadequate perfusion and atelectasis in inadequate ventilation.

Best practice – arterial blood gas analysis

Consider the patient's clinical history and physical examination

Systematically analyse the results

Integrate the clinical findings with interpretation of the data

---

Classification of imbalance

There are four classifications of imbalance with or without compensation:

- *respiratory* acidosis;
- *metabolic* acidosis;
- *respiratory* alkalosis;
- *metabolic* alkalosis.

Respiratory acidosis

Respiratory acidosis is caused by inadequate ventilation leading to the retention of carbon dioxide and an increase in free hydrogen ions.

Predisposing factors include:

- exacerbation of chronic obstructive pulmonary disease;
- pulmonary oedema;
- pneumonia;
- mechanical disruption to ventilation, e.g. diagphramatic rupture, fractured sternum;
- neurological disorder, e.g. intracranial events and neuro-muscular disorders;
- over sedation, i.e. opiates or sedatives;
- self poisoning.

An example of respiratory acidosis without metabolic compensation

pH 7.24
PCO_2 8.0
PO_2 8.7
HCO_3 24
BE 0
SaO_2 93%

It is vital that there is a fine balance between acids and bases to provide the optimum neutral environment for cell function. In the above example, the buffer system provided by the kidneys should counterbalance the free H^+ ions produced by the excessive CO_2. Compensation for acidosis or alkalosis is achieved by the other system (i.e. the kidneys will compensate for respiratory derangement and the lungs for metabolic derangement). The lungs however, provide a much quicker compensatory mechanism than the kidneys which can take hours or even days to compensate adequately.

An example of respiratory acidosis with metabolic compensation

pH 7.37
PCO_2 7.9
PO_2 9.6
HCO_3 32

BE +6
SaO$_2$ 95%

In this example there is an increase in the amount of HCO$_3$ reabsorbed by the kidneys to act as a buffer for the excessive free H+ ions. The compensation is only said to be adequate if the pH has returned to within normal limits, as in this example.

Metabolic acidosis

This involves excess fixed acid production, i.e. lactate or loss of HCO$_3$. Causes include:

- diarrhoea;
- cardiac arrest;
- diabetic ketoacidosis;
- renal failure;
- distributive shock;
- salicylate poisoning.

Example of metabolic acidosis without respiratory compensation

pH 7.20
PCO$_2$ 4.7
PO$_2$ 10.0
HCO$_3$ 16
BE −12
SaO$_2$ 96%

Here the lack of HCO$_3$ has resulted in a metabolic acidosis.

Example of metabolic acidosis with respiratory compensation

pH 7.35
PCO$_2$ 2.7
PO$_2$ 11.8
HCO$_3$ 12
BE −14

SaO_2 97%
B

Respiratory alkalosis
Respiratory alkalosis is caused by the over excretion of CO_2 leading to a reduction in free hydrogen ions and an alkalotic state. Predisposing factors include:

- hyperventilation in hysteria;
- over mechanical ventilation.

Example of respiratory alkalosis without metabolic compensation

pH 7.50
PCO_2 2.5
PO_2 8.6
HCO_3 22
BE +1
SaO_2 92%

Example of respiratory alkalosis with metabolic compensation

pH 7.44
PCO_2 2.6
PO_2 8.9
HCO_3 15
BE –9
SaO_2 93%

The patient excretes bicarbonate ions via the renal system in order to reduce the presence of alkaline buffers in the blood further.

Metabolic alkalosis
Metabolic alkalosis is caused by a loss of acids or an increase in alkaline buffers, i.e. bicarbonate. Causes include:

- gastrointestinal disorders, e.g. severe vomiting;
- overdose of antacids;
- diuretics.

An example of metabolic alkalosis without respiratory compensation

pH 7.67
PCO_2 4.2
PO_2 13.1
HCO_3 38
BE +15
SaO_2 98%

An example of metabolic alkalosis with respiratory compensation

pH 7.45
PCO_2 7.6
PO_2 12.4
HCO_3 32
BE +4
SaO_2 96%

The respiratory system retains CO_2 in order to create more available free hydrogen ions to balance the excess alkaline production, thereby maintaining the equilibrium.

MONITORING PRIORITIES OF A VENTILATED PATIENT

As intermittent positive pressure ventilation (IPPV) is totally converse to normal physiological breathing, on-going monitoring is essential. During spontaneous breathing air is 'sucked in' under a negative pressure whereas in IPPV air is delivered under a positive pressure.

There are many physical, as well as psychological, parameters to be monitored, all of which must be fully understood by the nurse caring for these patients. The primary physiological changes taking place concern the cardiovascular system. IPPV increases intrathoracic pressure which will impede venous return, reduce cardiac filling and reduce cardiac output. In addition, the fall in cardiac output leading to a reduction in renal blood flow stimulates the release of antidiuretic hormone (ADH) causing fluid retention and oedema.

There are two main categories of IPPV: *volume cycled* and *pressure cycled*. Volume cycled ventilation is rate set, volume set, pressure variable: i.e. the peak inspiratory pressure reached at each breath is dependent on the compliance of the lungs. This mode enables a preset volume to be delivered at a preset rate at the lowest pressure possible.

Pressure cycled ventilation is rate set, pressure set, volume variable: i.e. the volume delivered at each preset pressure is dependent on compliance. This mode avoids unnecessarily high peak airway pressures, reducing the risk of barotrauma, particularly in those at risk, e.g. acute lung injury.

Parameters to be monitored during IPPV

During intermittent positive pressure ventilation careful note should be taken of the following measurements.

- *Tidal volume (V_T)*: volume of air per expired breath. It should be the same or slightly more than the preset V_T. Aim for 6–8 ml/kg, i.e. maximum for a 70 kg person should be 560 ml per ventilation. A decrease in mortality has been demonstrated with patients with acute lung injury using these lower tidal volumes (Brower *et al*. 2000). If the inspired V_T does not correlate with the expired V_T in volume cycled ventilation, check for leaks in the circuit, check that the cuff on the endotracheal tube is inflated sufficiently and check the ventilator (inner valves, etc.). If tidal volume (V_T) is high, the patient is probably breathing spontaneously. Another cause of a high tidal volume is a nebuliser in the circuit.
- *Minute volume (mv)*: amount exhaled each minute. It should always be the same as preset minute volume (rate × V_T = mv).
- *Peak inspiratory pressure*: peak pressure at which the tidal volume is delivered. Measured in cmH_2O, it must always be at the lowest possible to ensure adequate ventilation. This will lessen the cardiovascular side-effects of IPPV and reduce the risks of barotrauma.

- *PEEP*: positive end expiratory pressure: this should range between +5 and +20 cmH$_2$O. PEEP facilitates a positive pressure at the end of expiration in the chest, promoting gaseous exchange at alveolar level. PEEP is over and above inspiratory pressure, i.e. if pressure is set at 20 cmH$_2$O and PEEP at 5 cm[12] the peak inspiratory pressure will be 25 cmH$_2$O.
- *FiO$_2$*: fraction of inspired O$_2$ expressed as a fraction of a whole, i.e. 40% = FiO$_2$ 0.40.

Monitoring the endotracheal tube

The following are key principles of the management of a patient with an endotracheal tube.

- Maintain patency: ventilation should be closely monitored and suction should be immediately available.
- Secure the end of the tube.
- Alter the position of the tube at the lips to prevent pressure ulceration.
- Document the length at which the tube is cut and tied and check regularly for migration from these markers.
- Ensure continuous pulse oximetry to detect hypoxaemia.
- Apply regular endotracheal suction, either with or without hyperinflation, to prevent sputum retention and maintain patency of the tube.
- Regularly auscultate for breath sounds to ensure equal inflation. The possibility of the tip of the tracheal tube slipping into the right main bronchus causing unilateral ventilation can therefore be excluded.
- Regular oral toilet, preferably with toothbrush and paste, will help to maintain oral hygiene.
- Secure/support ventilator tubing to prevent excess weight on the endotracheal tube.
- Check emergency equipment, i.e. intubation equipment, suction and manual re-breathe circuits at least once a shift in case of accidental extubation.
- Use endotracheal tubes with high volume, low pressure cuffs to minimise the risk of tracheal stenosis/ischaemia.

The nurse should be alert to the possible complications of endotracheal intubation. The acronym DOPE is helpful in detecting problems:

Displacement of tube
Obstruction of tube
Pneumothorax
Equipment

Other complications of tracheal intubation include oeso-phageal or right main bronchus intubation, herniation of the cuff, damage to vocal cords, tracheal stenosis, tracheal ulcera-tion, damage to soft palate and lips.

PRINCIPLES OF MONITORING A PATIENT WITH A CHEST DRAIN

A chest drain can be used to manage a variety of thoracic con-ditions. It can safely remove air (pneumothorax) or fluid (haemothorax, pleural effusion) from the pleural cavity and prevent its reintroduction, allowing the lungs to re-expand (Welch 1993).

The drain insertion site is determined by whether air or fluid requires removal. Air usually rises to the apex of the lung and is therefore most efficiently removed when the tip of the drain is anterior and apical to the chest cavity (Avery 2000). On the other hand fluid usually collects at the base of the lung and is therefore most efficiently removed when the drain is posterior and basal to the chest cavity (Graham 1996).

When monitoring a patient with a chest drain the following precautions should be observed.

- Monitor the patient's vital signs, in particular in relation to the patient's respiratory status.
- Request a chest X-ray following insertion of chest drain to check its position and ensure the lung has re-inflated.
- Administer prescribed analgesia for pain (Miller & Harvey 1993).
- Secure the drain to prevent movement, although care

should be taken if using tape because the connection can become disconnected without the practitioner noticing, resulting in air entering the chest cavity undetected (Godden & Hiley 1998).

- Regularly check the fluid level, as an underwater sealed drain operates as a one way valve allowing air to bubble out through the water during expiration and coughing but not permitting air to be drawn back in (Avery 2000).

- Observe and record the amount, consistency and colour of any drainage. If drainage is collecting in a fluid-dependent loop of the tubing either reposition or shorten the tube to prevent it from occurring (preferable) or regularly lift and drain the tubing (Schmelz *et al.* 1999).

- Observe the level of water in the tubing. It should fluctuate with respirations; a gradual decrease in fluctuation could indicate re-expansion of the lung while a sudden decrease suggests that the tube is blocked (Avery 2000). Bubbling is another sign that air is being evacuated from the pleural space; it should decrease as the lung re-inflates, if it doesn't there may be a leak in the patient's lung (Carroll 1991) – also check that there are no loose connections in the system. If a blocked tube is suspected, check that the cause is not a kinked tube. The tubing may need to be replaced. 'Milking' the tube is not recommended as this may suck lung tissue into the chest drain (Welch 1993).

- Monitor any suction used; low grade suction can be used to help remove air or fluid from the chest cavity. However insufficient suction will prevent lung expansion increasing the risk of tension pneumothorax (Avery 2000) while too much suction can lead to air and oxygen being 'sucked out' leading to hypoxia (Tang *et al.* 1999). A suction pressure of 10–20 cm H_2O is normally used (McManus 1998) NB: if a chest drain is connected to a suction unit which has been switched off it is equivalent to it being clamped off and could therefore result in a tension pneumothorax (Mallett & Dougherty 2000).

- Clamp the drain close to the chest wall only when changing the bottle/container or after accidental disconnection; the clamps should be removed as soon as possible (Brandt *et al.* 1994) because a build up of pressure can lead to a tension pneumothorax (Pierce 1995).
- Ensure the drainage bottle is kept below the level of the patient's chest to prevent fluid re-entering the pleural space (Avery 2000).
- Monitor the chest drain insertion site for indications of infection.

SCENARIOS

Scenario 1: Type 1 respiratory failure

Damien, a 22-year-old man weighing 65 kg, was involved in a motorcycle accident in which he was in collision with a car. On clinical and radiological examination in A+E he was found to have fractured ribs: 5th, 6th, 7th and 8th on the right side and 4th on the left causing a flail segment with paradoxical chest movements.

BP 90/60, pulse 100, respirations 36, core temperature 35.8°C. He was commenced on humidified O_2 via a facemask at 40%. Continuous ECG monitoring and pulse oximetry were also commenced. Blood was taken for a full biochemical, haematological screen, group and save and blood gas analysis:

pH 7.37

PCO_2 4.0

PO_2 5.5

HCO_3 24

BE −1

SaO_2 85%

What do these results tell you?

Despite the insertion of a thoracic epidural for pain control, Damien continued progress into severe Type 1 respiratory failure and was electively ventilated. Following ventilation and stabilisation a spinal CT scan was performed to exclude spinal injury. He was then transferred to ICU. Sedation and analgesia were provided with midazolam and a thoracic epidural. IPPV commenced at:

V_T: 455 ml (calculated at 6–8 ml/kg)

Rate: 12 breaths per minute

FiO_2: 7

PEEP: 7

Arterial blood gas analysis was repeated.

pH 7.44

PCO_2 3.8

PO_2 10.5

HCO_3 24

BE −2

SaO_2 96%

What do these results tell you?

With ventilation came an improvement in his blood gases on 70% O_2. Sedation was titrated not only to ensure adequate ventilation, but also so that Damien could be roused by voice and was able to communicate using non-verbal methods. This enabled staff to measure the efficacy of the epidural using a visual analogue pain rating scale and allay his anxieties through orientating him to his environment and circumstances.

On day 5 Damien was successfully weaned from ventilation and extubated. The thoracic epidural continued to provide excellent analgesia for his flail segment and spontaneous respiration (with supplementary humidified oxygen) did not present any difficulties. He was discharged from ICU after seven days.

Scenario 2: Type 2 respiratory failure

A 67-year-old man with a known history of emphysema presented with increasing breathlessness after a 'flu like' illness with purulent sputum and a fever.

On admission to A+E he was acutely breathless, centrally cyanosed and drowsy. Blood gas analysis was:

pH 7.11

PCO_2 10.8

PO_2 6.8

HCO_3 29

BE +5

SaO_2 84%

What do these results tell you?

A CXR demonstrated a right middle lobe collapse. He was commenced on O_2 at 40% and venous access was established with isotonic fluids at 100 ml/h. Because of the purulent sputum he was commenced on cefotaxime IV and regular bronchodilators. A urinary catheter was passed. At this time he was considered suitable for admission to a respiratory medical ward. He was reviewed one hour later and blood gases taken.

pH 7.10

PCO_2 11.1

PO_2 7.3

HCO_3 29

BE +5

SaO_2 85%

What do these results tell you?

The increase in PCO_2 indicated that the patient's condition might be deteriorating. In view of his past chronic medical history, his use of domicilary oxygen and the progressive nature of emphysema, it was decided that he was not a suitable candidate for invasive ventilation. He was therefore commenced on non-invasive ventilation (biphasic positive airway pressure ventilation (BIPAP)) via a nasal mask. During BIPAP the patient continued to breathe spontaneously but was assisted by the ventilator. In effect this is pressure support with positive end expiratory pressure (PEEP). This increases tidal volume (VT) and promotes alveolar gas exchange resulting in a reduction in the work of breathing and an improvement in gas exchange. This non-invasive method is a simpler alternative, avoiding the significant risks associated with invasive ventilation, e.g. cardiovascular instability. Within two hours the patient was showing improvement:

pH 7.19

PCO_2 9.0

PO_2 7.9

HCO_3 28

BE +4

SaO_2 88%

He continued to receive BIPAP for the next three days and with the aid of antibiotics, diuretics and physiotherapy was able to return home without the need for an ICU admission.

Scenario 3 Type 2 respiratory failure

A 22-year-old man, suffering from Duyenne's muscular dystrophy, was admitted to an acute medical ward with a chest infection. On admission he was anxious, but co-operative. Oxygen 40% was being administered via a face mask. BP was 120/80, HR is 100, respiratory rate is 26 and SpO_2 is 96%. He was being treated with broad spectrum antibiotics and a dextrose saline infusion was commenced at 100 ml per hour.

Six hours later he became progressively more drowsy and difficult to rouse. His respiratory effort remained unchanged and his SpO_2 was 97%. He looked flushed but was apyrexial. Arterial blood gas results were as follows:

pH 7.21

PCO_2 10.6

PO_2 9.6

HCO_2 22

BE +1

SaO_2 97%

What do these results tell you?

The PCO_2 is high and the patient has respiratory acodosis, requiring urgent ICU referral. This example demonstrates one limitation of pulse oximetry: a normal SpO_2 does not necessarily correlate with adequate ventilation.

CONCLUSION

Monitoring respiratory function requires accurate assessment of the efficacy of breathing, work of breathing and adequacy of ventilation together with a comprehensive patient assessment. Peak expiratory flow rate measurements, pulse oximetry and arterial blood gas analysis also contribute to the monitoring process.

REFERENCES

Adam, S. & Osborne, S. (1997) *Critical Care Nursing: Science and Practice*. Oxford University Press.

Athern, J., Fildes, S. & Peters, R. (1995) A guide to blood gases. *Nursing Standard* **9** (49), 50–52.

Avery, S. (2000) Insertion and management of chest drains. *Nursing Times Plus* **96** (37), 3–6.

Berge, K.H., Lanier, W.L., Scanlon, P.D. (1988) Ischaemic digital skin necrosis: a complication of the reusable nelcor pulse oximeter probe. *Anesthesia and Analgesia* **67**, 712–713.

Blackwell, B. (1998) The practice and perception of intensive care staff using the closed suctioning system. *Journal of Advances in Nursing* **28** (5), 1020–1029.

Brandt, M. *et al*. (1994) The paediatric chest tube. *Clinical Intensive Care* **5** (3), 123–129.

Brewis, R.A. (1996) *Respiratory Medicine*. W.B. Saunders, Philadelphia.

Brocke-Utne (1992) Perioperative corneal abrasions *Anaesthesiology* **77**, 221.

Brower, R., Matthay, M., Morris, A. *et al*. (2000) Ventilation with lower tidal volumes as compared with traditional tidal volumes for acute lung injury and the acute respiratory distress syndrome. *New England Journal of Medicine* **342** (18), 1301–1308.

Brower, R., Shanholtz, C., Fessler, H. *et al*. (1999) Prospective RCT comparing traditional vs reduced VT ventilation in acute respiratory distress syndrome patients. *Critical Care Medicine* **27** (8), 1492–1498.

Carroll, P. (1991) What's new in chest tube management. *Registered Nurse* **54** (5), 35–40.

Carroll, P. (1998) Preventing noscomial pneumonia. *Registered Nurse* **61** (6), 44–48.

Coleman, M.D. & Coleman, N.A. (1996) Drug induced methaemglobinaemia: Treatment issues. *Drug Safety* **14** (6), 394–405.

Comroe, J.H. & Botelho, S. (1947) The unreliability of cyanosis in the recognition of arterial anoxaemia. *American Journal of Medical Science* **214**, 1–5.

Cote, C.J., Goldstein, A., Fuchsman, W.H. *et al*. (1988) The effect of nail polish on pulse oximetry. *Anesthesia and Analgesia* **67**, 683–686.

Davidson, J.A. & Hosie, H.E. (1993) Limitations of pulse oximetry: respiratory insufficiency – a failure of detection. *British Medical Journal* **307** (6900), 372–373.

Dobson, F. (1993) Shedding light on pulse oximetry. *Nursing Standard* **7** (46), 4–11.

Driscoll, P., Brown, T., Gwinnutt, C. *et al*. (1997) *A Simple Guide to Blood Gas Analysis*. BMJ Publishing Group, London.

Godden, J. & Hiley, C. (1998) Managing the patient with a chest drain: a review. *Nursing Standard* **12** (32), 35–39.

Graham, A. (1996) Chest drain insertion. 'How to' Guide Series *Care of the Critically Ill* **12** (5).

Hanning, C.D. & Alexander-Williams, J.M. (1995) Pulse oximetry: a practical review. *British Medical Journal* **311**, 367–370.

Harrahill, M. (1991) Pulse oximetry, pearls and pitfalls. *Journal of Emergency Nursing* **17** (6), 437–439.

Hinds, C.J. & Watson, D. (1996) *Intensive Care, a concise textbook* 2nd edn. W.B. Saunders, London.

Hubbard & Mechan (1997) The Physiology of Health and Illness with Related Anatomy. Stanley Thorn, Cheltenham.

Hutton, P. & Clutton-Brock, T. (1993) The benefits and pitfalls of pulse oximetry. *British Medical Journa* **307**, 457–458.

Jenson, L.A., Onyskiw, J.E. & Prasad, N.G.N. (1998) Meta-analysis of arterial oxygenation saturation monitoring by pulse oximetry in adults. *Heart and Lung* **27** (6), 387–408.

Jevon, P. & Ewens, B. (2000) Pulse oximetry. *Nursing Times* **96** (26), 43–44.

Jevon, P., Ewens, B. & Manzie, J. (2000) Peak flow. *Nursing Times* **96** (38), 49–50.

Jevon, P. & Ewens, B. (2001) Assessment of a breathless patient. *Nursing Standard* **15** (16), 48–53.

Johnson, N. (1987) *Respiratory Medicine*. Blackwell Scientific Publications, Oxford.

Law, C. (2000) A guide to assessing sputum *Nursing Times* **96** (24), Respiratory Care Supplement **7–10**.

Lowton, K. (1999) Pulse oximeters for the detection of hypoxaemia. *Professional Nurse* **14** (5), 343–350.

Lynne, M., Scnapp, M.D., Neal, H. *et al.* (1990) Pulse oximetry: uses and abuses. *Chest* **98**, 1244–1250.

Mackreth, B. (1990) Assessing pulse oximetry in the field. *Journal of Emergency Medical Services* **15**, 56–57, 59–60.

Mallett, J. & Dougherty, L. (2000), eds *The Royal Marsden Hospital Manual of Clinical Nursing Procedures*. Blackwell Science, Oxford.

McManus, K. (1998) Chest drainage systems. 'How to' Guide Series *Care of the Critically Ill* **14** (4).

Middleton, S. & Middleton, P.G. (1998) Assessment. In: Pryor, J.A. & Webber, B.A., eds *Physiotherapy for Respiratory and Cardiac Problems*. Churchill Livingstone, Edinburgh.

Miller, A. & Harvey, J. (1993) Guidelines for the management of spontaneous pneumothorax. Standards of Care Committee, British Thoracic Society. *British Medical Journal* **307** (6896), 114–117.

Nunn, A.J. & Gregg, I. (1989) New regression equations for predicting peak expiratory flow in adults. *British Medical Journal* **298**, 1068–1070.

Partridge, M. (1997) *Asthma Care; a guide to peak flow*. Allen & Hanburys, Uxbridge.

Pierce, L. (1995) *Guide to Mechanical Ventilation and Intensive Respiratory Care*. W.B. Saunders, London.

Place, B. (1998) Pulse oximetry in adults. *Nursing Times* **94** (50), 48–49.

Place, B. (2000) Pulse oximetry: benefits and limitations. *Nursing Times* **96** (26), 42.

Ralston, A.C. *et al*. (1991) Potential errors in pulse oximetry. *Anaesthesia* **46** (4), 291–295.

Rees, J. & Price, J.F. (1999). *ABC of Asthma*. BMJ Books, London.

Resuscitation Council UK (2000). *Advanced Life Support Manual* 4th edn. Resuscitation Council UK, London.

Reynolds, K.J. *et al*. (1993) The effect of dyshemoglobins on pulse oximetry: Part 1, Theoretical approach & Part 2, Experimental results using an *in vitro* test system. *Journal of Clinical Monitoring* **9** (2), 81–90.

Richardson, N.G.B. & Hale, J.E. (1995) Pulse oximetry – an unusual complication. *British Journal of Intensive Care* **5**(10), 326–327.

Ross-Plummer, B. (2000) Preparing patients with asthma for discharge. *Nursing Times* **96**, 24 Ntplus 13–15.

Schmelz, J. *et al*. (1999) Effects of position of chest drainage tube on volume drained and pressure. *American Journal of Critical Care* **8** (5), 319–323.

Schnapp, L.M. & Cohen, N.H. (1990) Pulse oximetry: uses and abuses. *Chest* **98**, 1244–1250.

Severinghaus, J.W. & Koh, S.O. (1990) Effect of anaemia on pulse oximetry accuracy at low saturation. *Journal of Clinical Monitoring* **6**, 85–88.

Shoulders-Odom, B. (2000) Using an algorithm to interpret arterial blood gases. *Dimensions of Critical Care Nursing* **19** (1), 36.

Smith, R. & Olson, M. (1989) Drug induced methaemoglobinaemia on pulse oximetry and mixed venous oximetry. *Anaesthesiology* **70**, 112–117.

Stoneham, M.D. *et al*. (1994) Knowledge about pulse oximetry amongst medical and nursing staff. *The Lancet* **344**, 1339–1342.

Tang, A. *et al*. (1999) A regional survey of chest drains: evidence-based practice? *Postgraduate Medical Journal* **75** (886), 471–474.

Technology Subcommittee of the Working Group on Critical Care (1992) Non-invasive blood gas monitoring: a review for use in the adult critical care unit. *Canadian Medical Association Journal* **146**, 703–712.

Thibodeau, G. & Patton, K. (1999). *Anatomy & Physiology*. Mosby, London.

Torrance, C. & Elley, K. (1997) Respiration, technique and observation 1. *Nursing Times* **43,** suppl.

Valenti, L., Tamblyn, R. & Rozinski, M.B. (1997) *Critical Care Nursing*. J B Lippincott, New York.

Wahr, J.A & Tremper, K.K. (1996) Oxygen measurement and monitoring techniques. In: C. Prys-Roberts & B.R. Brown Jr, eds *International Practice of Anaesthesia*. Butterworth Heinemann, Oxford.

Welch, J. (1993) Chest drains and pleural drainage. *Surgical Nurse* **6** (5), 7–12.

Weston Smith, S.G.W., Glass, U.H., Acharya, J. *et al.* (1989) Pulse oximetry in sickle cell disease. *Clinical and Laboratory Haematology* **11**, 185–188.

Woodrow, P. (1999) Pulse oximetry. *Nursing Standard* **13** (42), 42–47.

2 | Monitoring Cardiovascular Function 1: ECG Monitoring

INTRODUCTION

ECG monitoring is one of the most valuable diagnostic tools in modern medicine. It is essential if disorders of the cardiac rhythm are to be recognised, and can help with diagnosis and alert healthcare staff to changes in a patient's condition.

However ECG monitoring must be meticulously undertaken. Consequences of poor technique include misinterpretation of arrhythmias, mistaken diagnosis, wasted investigations and mismanagement of the patient. Nurses must understand the principles of ECG monitoring, including troubleshooting, and recognition of important arrhythmias.

The aim of this chapter is to understand the principles of ECG monitoring.

LEARNING OBJECTIVES

At the end of the chapter the reader will be able to:

❑ describe the common features of a *cardiac monitor*;
❑ describe how to set up *ECG monitoring*;
❑ discuss the potential *problems* that may be encountered with ECG monitoring;
❑ describe the *ECG* and its *relation to cardiac contraction*;
❑ describe a systematic approach to *ECG interpretation*;
❑ define and classify *cardiac arrhythmias*;
❑ *recognise* important cardiac arrhythmias.

COMMON FEATURES OF A CARDIAC MONITOR

The bedside cardiac monitor (Fig. 2.1) or oscilloscope provides a continuous display of the patient's ECG and has the following common features.

- *Screen for displaying the ECG trace*: a dull/bright switch can be adjusted if the ECG recording and background is too light or too dark.
- *ECG printout facility*: this is particularly useful for recording cardiac arrhythmias and is invaluable for both diagnostic and treatment purposes. The ECG printouts can also complement the patient's records.
- *Heart rate counter*: most calculate the heart rate by counting the number of QRS complexes in a minute.
- *Monitor alarms*: can alert the nurse to changes in the heart rate that are outside preset limits. If the monitor alarms are

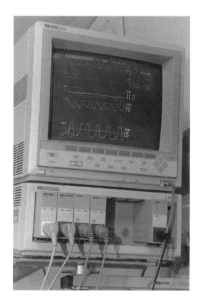

Fig. 2.1 Bedside cardiac monitor

to be relied upon, they should be on and set within safe parameters (agreed locally) and based on the patient's clinical condition. More advanced monitors can identify important cardiac arrhythmias and alarm accordingly.

- *Lead select switch*: lead II is usually the most popular lead for ECG monitoring.
- *ECG gain*: this can alter the gain or size of the ECG complex; if it is set too low or too high the ECG trace may be unclear and misinterpreted.

SETTING UP ECG MONITORING

The following measures should be observed when setting up ECG monitoring.

(1) Explain the procedure to the patient.
(2) Prepare the skin: ensure it is dry prior to attaching the ECG electrodes. If necessary shave off any excess hair (Perez 1996a). This will also make it less uncomfortable for the patient when the electrodes are removed.
(3) Attach the electrodes following locally agreed guidelines. Switch the cardiac monitor on and select the required monitoring lead.
(4) Ensure the ECG trace is clear. Rectify any difficulties encountered (see below).
(5) Ensure alarms are set within safe parameters following locally agreed guidelines and according to the patient's clinical condition.
(6) Ensure the cardiac monitor can clearly be seen.
(7) Document in the patient's notes that ECG monitoring has commenced.

Adapted from Jevon 2000

Correct electrode placement (Fig. 2.2) is crucial for obtaining accurate information from any monitoring lead (Jacobson 2000). The electrode placement and monitoring lead selected for ECG monitoring will depend on the factors listed below.

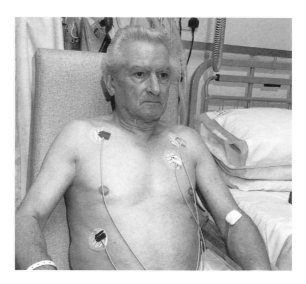

Fig. 2.2 Suggested ECG electrode placement using a 5 wire monitoring system

- *Monitoring system* (e.g. 3 or 5 wire monitoring system). If a 5 wire system is being used a suggested ECG electrode placement is red (right shoulder), yellow (left shoulder), green (left lower thorax/hip region), black (right lower thorax/hip region) and white on the chest in the desired V position, usually V1 (Jacobson 2000). If a 3 wire system is being used a suggested ECG electrode placement is red (right shoulder), yellow (left shoulder) and green (left lower thorax/hip region).
- *Goals of monitoring*, e.g. if arrhythmia diagnosis is the goal.
- *Patient's clinical situation* (Jacobson 2000): e.g. in cardio-pulmonary resuscitation, the precordium should be left unobstructed in case defibrillation is required (Resuscitation Council UK 2000).

NB: ECG monitoring should *complement not replace* basic nursing observations of the patient. Treat the patient not the monitor.

POTENTIAL PROBLEMS WITH ECG MONITORING

There are many problems that can occur with ECG monitoring, some are due to the limitations of the monitoring system itself while others are due to poor technique (Meltzer *et al.* 1977). Potential problems that may be encountered include the following.

The 'flat line' trace

Check the patient immediately. However, the most likely cause is mechanical. Check that the:

- correct monitoring lead is selected (usually lead 11);
- ECG gain is set correctly;
- electrodes are 'in-date' and that the gel sponge is moist, not dry;
- electrodes are properly connected;
- leads are plugged into the monitor.

Poor quality ECG trace

If the ECG trace quality is poor, check:

- all the connections;
- the brightness display;
- that the electrodes are 'in-date' and that the gel sponge is moist, not dry (Perez 1996a);
- that the electrodes are properly attached.

If there are still difficulties obtaining a clear ECG trace, wiping the skin with an alcohol wipe may help. If the patient is sweating profusely the application of a small amount of tincture benzoin to the skin, leaving it to dry before applying the electrodes, is recommended (Jowett & Thompson 1995). As electrodes tend to dry out after about three days, they should be changed at least that often though every 24h may be optimum to maintain skin integrity (Perez 1996b).

Interference and artifacts

Poor electrode contact, patient movement and electrical interference, e.g. from bedside infusion pumps, can cause a 'fuzzy' appearance on the ECG trace. Interference can be minimised by applying the electrodes over bone rather than muscle (Resuscitation Council UK 2000). The patient should also be reassured and kept warm.

Wandering baseline

A wandering baseline (ECG trace going up and down) is usually caused by patient movement or simply by respiration. If respiration is the cause and the problem is not transient, re-positioning of the electrodes away from the lower ribs is advisable (Meltzer *et al.* 1977).

Small ECG complexes

Sometimes the ECG complexes may be too small and unrecognisable. Possible causes include pericardial effusion, obesity and hypothyroidism. However sometimes it can be caused by a technical problem. Check that the ECG gain is correctly set and lead 11 is being monitored. Repositioning the electrodes or selecting another monitoring lead sometimes helps.

Incorrect heart rate display

If the ECG complexes are too small, a false low heart rate may be displayed. Large T waves, muscle movement and interference can be mistaken for QRS complexes resulting in a false high heart rate being displayed. The nurse must be alert to the possibility of inaccurate heart rate readings, which can in particular be caused by poor electrode contact and interference

(Ren *et al.* 1998). To minimise the potential for inaccuracies, a reliable good quality ECG trace should be obtained.

Skin irritation

ECG electrodes can cause skin irritation. The electrode sites should be regularly examined and if the patient's skin appears irritated select another electrode placement (Paul & Hebra 1998).

False alarms

Frequent false alarms will undermine the rationale for setting alarms and can also cause undue anxiety for the patient. It is important to ensure that the alarms are correctly and sensibly set and that the ECG is accurate, reliable and of a high standard.

Best practice – ECG monitoring

Ensure adequate skin preparation

Use ECG electrodes that are in date, with moist gel sponge

Position ECG electrodes and select monitoring lead following locally agreed protocols

Set cardiac monitor alarms according to the patient's clinical condition

Ensure the ECG trace is accurate

Ensure the cardiac monitor is visible

THE ECG AND ITS RELATION TO CARDIAC CONTRACTION (FIG. 2.3)

The ECG functions in four stages as follows.

(1) The sinus node fires and the electrical impulse spreads across the atria. This results in atrial contraction (P wave).

(2) On arriving at the AV junction the impulse is delayed, allowing the atria time to contract fully and eject blood into the ventricles. This brief period of absent electrical activ-

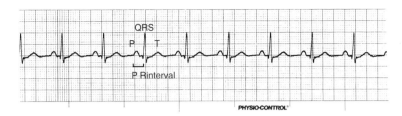

Fig. 2.3 The ECG and its relation to cardiac contraction (PQRST complex)

ity is represented on the ECG by a straight (isoelectric) line between the end of the P wave and the beginning of the QRS complex. The PR interval represents atrial depolarisation and the impulse delay in the AV junction prior to ventricular depolarisation.

(3) The impulse is then conducted down to the ventricles through the bundle of His, right and left bundle branches and Purkinje fibres causing ventricular depolarisation and contraction (QRS complex).

(4) The ventricles then repolarise (T wave).

SYSTEMATIC APPROACH TO ECG INTERPRETATION

The following systematic approach to ECG interpretation enables the practitioner to interpret most ECG traces and arrive at a reliable diagnosis on which to base effective treatment. The five-stage approach is as follows:

• QRS rate;
• QRS rhythm;
• P waves;
• relationship between P waves and QRS complexes;
• QRS width.

QRS rate

Estimate the QRS rate by counting the number of large (1 cm) squares between adjacent QRS complexes and dividing it into 300, e.g. the QRS rate in Fig. 2.3 is approximately 80 (300/3.8) (Perez 1996a).

Normal ventricular rate is 60–100 beats/min
Bradycardia – rate <60
Tachycardia – rate >100

If the QRS rhythm is irregular it is preferable to estimate the rate by counting the number of complexes in a 15 second ECG strip and then multiplying it by 4.

QRS rhythm

Determine whether the QRS rhythm is regular or irregular. If it is irregular, establish if there is a common pattern or whether it is very erratic. Causes of an irregular QRS rhythm include sinus arrhythmia, atrial fibrillation, premature complexes and some atrioventricular blocks.

P waves

Determine whether P waves are present. They should be upright in lead 11 and be all of the same morphology. P waves of different morphology indicate a changing atrial pacemaker. P waves may be absent in some conduction disturbances and sometimes they may be difficult to distinguish or indeed be 'hidden' in the QRS in some tachyarrhythmias.

Relationship between the P waves and the QRS complexes

If P waves are present, determine whether they precede each QRS complex. Calculate the PR interval: it should remain constant and the normal range is 3–5 small squares. A shortened or prolonged PR interval is indicative of a conduction abnormality. Sometimes there can be complete dissociation between the P waves and QRS complexes, e.g. third degree heart block.

QRS width

Calculate the QRS width. It should be <2.5 small squares. Causes of a wide QRS include bundle branch block, ventricular premature contractions and ventricular tachycardia.

Sinus rhythm

This is illustrated in Fig. 2.4.

QRS rate: 80
QRS rhythm: regular
P waves: present and normal
Relationship between P waves and QRS: the P waves precede each QRS and the PR interval is normal
QRS width: normal (<2.5 squares)

The impulse originates in the sinus node at a rate of between 60 and 100 beats/min, is regular and is conducted down the normal pathways and with no abnormal delays, i.e. sinus rhythm.

Best practice – ECG interpretation:

Assess the patient for adverse signs

Calculate the QRS rate

Ascertain the QRS rhythm

Identify if P waves are present

Assess the relationship between P waves and QRS complexes

Calculate the QRS width

Obtain 12 lead ECG if necessary

DEFINITION AND CLASSIFICATION OF CARDIAC ARRHYTHMIAS

A 'cardiac arrhythmia' can be defined as any ECG rhythm that deviates from normal sinus rhythm.

Cardiac arrhythmias can be classified into one of two groups (Meltzer *et al.* 1977):

- arrhythmias resulting from a disturbance in impulse *formation*;
- arrhythmias resulting from a disturbance in impulse *conduction*.

NB: some cardiac arrhythmias may have a disturbance in both impulse formation and impulse conduction.

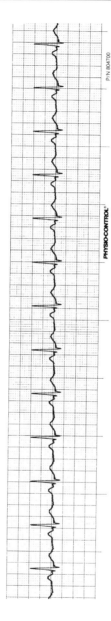

Fig. 2.4 Sinus rhythm

Arrhythmias resulting from a disturbance in impulse formation

These arrhythmias can be classified in respect of their site of origin and the mechanism of the disturbance as shown below (adapted from Jevon 2000).

Site of origin

The following features are significant:

- *SA node*: sinus rhythms, e.g. sinus bradycardia, sinus tachycardia;
- *atria*: atrial rhythms, e.g. atrial premature, atrial fibrillation;
- *AV junction*: junctional rhythms, e.g. junction rhythm;
- *ventricles*: ventricular rhythms, e.g. ventricular premature beats, ventricular tachycardia.

Mechanism

Features arising from the mechanism of the disturbance are:

- tachycardia >100 beats/minute;
- bradycardia <60 beats/minute;
- premature contractions;
- flutter;
- fibrillation.

Arrhythmias resulting from a disturbance in impulse conduction

A disturbance in conduction relates to an abnormal delay or block of the impulse at any point along the conduction system. They are traditionally categorised according to the site of the defect:

- *sinoatrial blocks*, e.g. sinus arrest;
- *atrioventricular* blocks, e.g. first, second, third degree block;
- *intraventricular blocks*, e.g. right and left bundle branch blocks.

RECOGNITION OF IMPORTANT ARRHYTHMIAS

When interpreting arrhythmias it is important to assess:

- the haemodynamic effect: clinical signs of a low cardiac output include hypotension, impaired consciousness, chest pain, dyspnoea and heart failure (European Resuscitation Council 1998);
- whether there is a risk of cardiac arrest.

Sinus tachycardia

This is illustrated in Fig. 2.5.

QRS rate: 120
QRS rhythm: regular
P waves: present and normal
Relationship between P waves and QRS complexes: P waves precede every QRS complex; PR interval normal
QRS width: normal

The ECG shows the same characteristics as sinus rhythm except that the ventricular (QRS) rate is >100 beats/min. It is abnormal and 'treatment' is generally aimed at identifying, and where appropriate, treating the cause.

Causes include anxiety, acute blood loss, anxiety, exercise, shock, pyrexia and drugs, e.g. hydralazine, nebulised salbutamol. Of greater importance is that it may be a manifestation of heart failure when it is a reflex mechanism to compensate for reduced stroke volume (Meltzer *et al.* 1977). Sometimes beta-blockers are prescribed with caution, e.g. in acute myocardial infarction.

Sinus bradycardia

Sinus brachycardia is illustrated in Fig. 2.6.

QRS rate: 40
QRS rhythm: regular
P waves: present and normal
Relationship between P waves and QRS complexes: P waves precede each QRS complex and the PR interval is normal
QRS width: normal

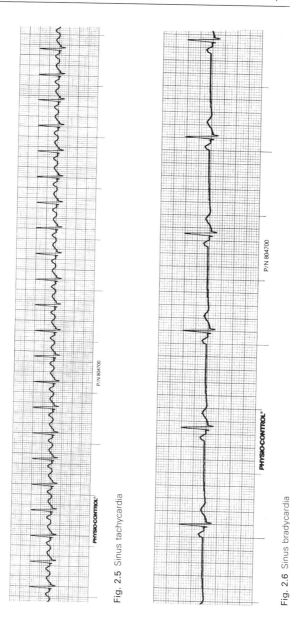

Fig. 2.5 Sinus tachycardia

Fig. 2.6 Sinus bradycardia

ECG shows the same characteristics as sinus rhythm except that the ventricular rate is <60 beats/min. Causes include vagal stimulation, e.g. during tracheal suction, increased intracranial pressure, hypoxia, severe pain, hypothermia and drugs, e.g. beta blockers. Sometimes it is normal for the patient, e.g. an athlete. Treatment often requires oxygen and atropine. Sometimes pacing may be indicated.

Atrial fibrillation
This is illustrated in Fig. 2.7.

QRS rate 140
QRS rhythm: irregular and very erratic
P waves: not present, irregular baseline – small, irregular and rapid oscillations
Relationship between P waves and QRS complexes: no P waves present
QRS width: normal

Atrial fibrillation is characterised by absent P waves, irregular baseline and irregular QRS complexes. The loss of atrial contraction or 'atrial kick' results in a 25% reduction in cardiac output. The ventricular rate can vary and treatment often includes digoxin. Cardioversion is sometimes required.

Atrial flutter
Fig. 2.8 illustrates atrial flutter.

QRS rate: 100
QRS rhythm: regular
P waves: flutter 'sawtooth' waves at a rate of 300 per minute
Relationship between P waves and QRS complexes: has no meaning and is not measured
QRS width: normal

Atrial flutter is characterised by the 'sawtooth' flutter waves which usually have a rate at approximately 300 per minute. The ventricular response depends on the degree of atrioven-

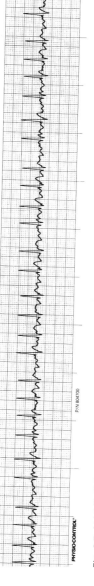

Fig. 2.7 Atrial fibrillation

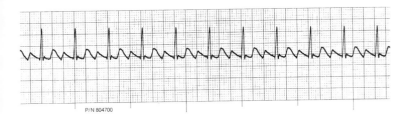

P/N 804700

Fig. 2.8 Atrial flutter

tricular block; in the example it is 3:1. Treatment could include digoxin or amiodarone. Cardioversion may be required.

Narrow complex tachycardia
The features of this are shown in Fig. 2.9.

QRS rate: 180
QRS rhythm: regular
P waves: unable to identify (situated on T waves?)
Relationship between P waves and QRS complexes: unable to determine
QRS width: normal

Unlike sinus tachycardia, narrow complex tachycardia (sometimes referred to as supraventricular tachycardia) starts and ends abruptly. The rate is always >140 beats per minute. A 12 lead ECG will help to determine the exact diagnosis. The key issue with this ECG is the QRS width, which rules out the often more serious broad complex (ventricular) tachycardia. Treatment, which will depend on how compromised the patient is, could include vagal manoeuvres, adenosine, amiodarone and cardioversion.

Broad complex tachycardia
Fig. 2.10 shows the salient features of broad complex tachycardia.

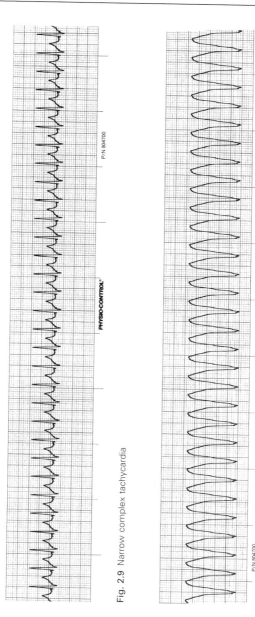

Fig. 2.9 Narrow complex tachycardia

Fig. 2.10 Broad complex tachycardia

QRS rate: 180
QRS rhythm: regular
P waves: not seen
Relationship between P waves and QRS complexes: unable to
    determine
QRS width: wide

Broad complex tachycardia usually results from a focus in the ventricles firing at a rapid rate. The patient may or may not lose cardiac output. The ECG shows a rapid heart rate usually over 150 per minute and the QRS complex is characteristically wide (>2.5 small squares). The ECG configuration can vary depending on where in the ventricles the focus is. If the patient has arrested the definitive treatment is rapid defibrillation. Other treatment could include drugs, e.g. lignocaine or amiodarone, and cardioversion.

Ventricular fibrillation

In ventricular fibrillation all coordination of electrical activity in the ventricular myocardium is lost, resulting in cardiac arrest. The ECG is characteristic, a bizarre irregular waveform apparently random in both frequency and amplitude. It can be classified as either coarse (Fig. 2.11) or fine (Fig. 2.12). Certainly the latter is significant in resuscitation because it can be mistaken for asystole, particularly if there is some interference. The definitive treatment is rapid defibrillation (Resuscitation Council UK 2000).

Asystole

Asystole (Fig. 2.13) is characteristically an undulating line and rarely a straight line.

In all cases of apparent asystole, the ECG trace should be viewed with suspicion before arrival at a final diagnosis. Check the patient. Other causes of a straight line ECG trace should be excluded, e.g. incorrect lead setting, disconnected leads and ECG gain incorrectly set. It is important not to miss ventricular fibrillation.

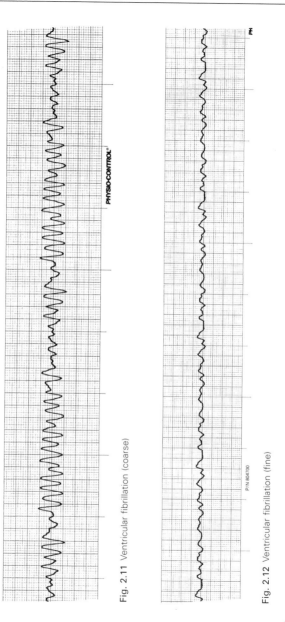

Fig. 2.11 Ventricular fibrillation (coarse)

Fig. 2.12 Ventricular fibrillation (fine)

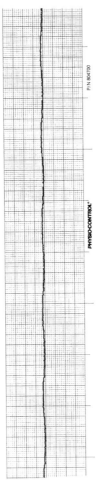

Fig. 2.13 Asystole

Pulseless electrical activity

Pulseless electrical activity (see Fig. 2.4) is a condition in which the patient is pulseless, but has a normal ECG trace. The diagnosis is made from a combination of the clinical absence of a cardiac output together with an ECG trace that would normally be associated with a good pulse.

Scenario

A 40-year-old man is admitted to the Coronary Care Unit with an acute inferior myocardial infarction. On admission BP is 120/90, pulse 70 sinus rhythm, resps 15 and temperature 36.7 degrees centigrade. The cardiac monitor starts to alarm as it has recognised 'asystole'. What would you do?

First of all check the patient. He is conscious, sitting up in bed and smiling. The cardiac monitor is still alarming 'asystole'. What would you do?

The ECG displays is a straight line, which the monitor has mistaken for asystole. There must be a mechanical problem. The lead select on the cardiac monitor is checked to ensure the desired lead has been selected. In addition the ECG gain (size) on the monitor is checked and is found to be fine. The leads are checked to ensure they are still connected. One of the leads has become disconnected from the electrode resulting in a straight line on the ECG. Following reconnection, sinus rhythm 70 BPM is displayed on the cardiac monitor.

CONCLUSION

ECG monitoring is central to the care of a critically ill patient. It must be meticulously undertaken in order to avoid misinterpretation of arrhythmias, mistaken diagnosis, wasted investigations and mismanagement of the patient. Nurses need to understand the principles of ECG monitoring, including trouble shooting and recognise important cardiac arrhythmias. Always remember to treat the patient not the monitor.

REFERENCES

European Resuscitation Council (1998) *European Resuscitation Council Guidelines for Resuscitation.* Elsevier, Oxford.

Jacobson, C. (2000) Optimum bedside cardiac monitoring. *Progress in Cardiovascular Nursing* **15** (4), 134–137.

Jevon, P. (2000) Cardiac monitoring. *Nursing Times* **96** (23), 43.

Jowett, N.I. & Thompson, D.R. (1995). *Comprehensive Coronary Care,* 2nd edn. Scutari Press/RCN, London.

Meltzer, L.E., Pinneo, R. & Kitchell, J.R. (1977) *Intensive Coronary Care, a Manual for Nurses* 3rd edn. Prentice-Hall, London.

Paul, S. & Hebra, J. (1998) *The Nurse's Guide to Cardiac Rhythm Interpretation.* W.B. Saunders. Philadelphia.

Perez, A. (1996a) Cardiac monitoring: mastering the essentials. *Registered Nurse* **59** (8), 32–39.

Perez, A. (1996b) EKG electrode placement: a refresher course. *Registered Nurse* **59** (9), 29–31.

Ren, Y., Yang, L. & Hu, P. (1998) Analysis of influencing factors on ECG monitoring. *Shanxi Nursing Journal* **12** (5), 213–214.

Resuscitation Council UK (2000). *Advanced Life Support Manual* 4th edn. Resuscitation Council UK, London.

Monitoring Cardiovascular Function 2: Haemodynamic Monitoring

3

INTRODUCTION

Haemodynamics can be defined as the study of the physical aspects of blood circulation, including cardiac function and peripheral vascular physiological characteristics (Mosby 1998). Haemodynamic monitoring is central to the care of a critically ill patient and can be classified as *non-invasive*, *invasive* and *derived* (i.e. data calculated from other measurements).

'Haemodynamic measurements are important to establish a precise diagnosis, determine appropriate therapy and monitor the response to that therapy' (Gomersall & Oh 1997). In particular they can assist in the early recognition of shock, where the immediate provision of circulatory support is paramount (Hinds & Watson 1999).

The aim of this chapter is to understand the principles of haemodynamic monitoring.

LEARNING OBJECTIVES

At the end of the chapter the reader will be able to:

❏ discuss the factors affecting *tissue perfusion*;
❏ define and classify *circulatory shock*;
❏ describe non-invasive methods of *haemodynamic monitoring*;
❏ outline the general principles of monitoring with *transducers*;
❏ discuss the principles of *central venous pressure monitoring*;
❏ outline and discuss the principles of *pulmonary artery pressure monitoring*;
❏ discuss the principles of *cardiac output studies*.

FACTORS AFFECTING TISSUE PERFUSION

Tissue perfusion is dependent upon an adequate blood pressure in the aorta. This pressure is determined by the product of two factors: *cardiac output* and *peripheral resistance* (Green 1991), see Fig. 3.1.

Cardiac output

Cardiac output = heart rate × stroke volume

Cardiac output is the amount of blood ejected from the left ventricle in one minute. At rest this is approximately 5000 ml. It is determined by heart rate and stroke volume.

Heart rate

Factors influencing heart rate include baroreceptor activity, the Bainbridge effect, pyrexia, higher centres, intracranial pressure and oxygen and carbon dioxide levels in the blood.

Stroke volume

Stroke volume is the amount of blood ejected from the left ventricle in one contraction. At rest this is approximately 70 ml. It is affected by heart rate, myocardial contractility, preload and afterload (Fig. 3.1).

- *Heart rate*: tachycardia reduces diastolic filling time resulting in a decreased stroke volume.
- *Myocardial contractility* refers to the ability of the heart to function independently of the changes in preload and after-

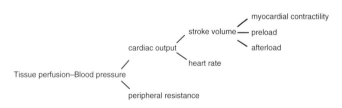

Fig. 3.1 Overview of factors affecting tissue perfusion.

Table. 3.1 Factors affecting myocardial contractility

Increased contractility:	drugs with inotropic properties, e.g. dobutamine, dopamine (dose related) digoxin, adrenaline, noradrenaline; circulating catecholamines; calcium; increased preload hyperthyroidism
Decreased contractility:	drugs with negative inotropic properties, e.g. lignocaine; hypoxia; hypocalcaemia and calcium channel blockers; beta adrenergic blockers, e.g. atenolol; decreased preload; functional deficit, e.g. following myocardial infarction

load (Hinds & Watson 1996). It is commonly referred to as the 'force of contraction'. Inotropic drugs, e.g. dobutamine, adrenaline, can increase myocardial contractility. Table 3.1 lists factors affecting myocardial contractility.

- *Preload* (or end diastolic volume/pressure) is the tension of the myocardial fibres at the end of diastole just before ventricular contraction (Hinds & Watson 1996). Starling's law of the heart states that 'the force of myocardial contraction is directly proportional to the initial fibre length', i.e. stretched fibres contract more forcefully (not overstretched). Venous return is the main factor determining preload and as the filling pressure rises, stroke volume increases. However in an overstretched ventricle, excessive dilatation may result in a fall in stroke volume.

  In the clinical setting manipulation of the preload is the most efficient method of improving cardiac output because it is associated with only a minimal rise in oxygen consumption (Hinds & Watson 1996). Table 3.2 lists factors affecting preload.

- *Afterload* is the resistance to the outflow of blood provided by the vasculature which must be overcome by the ventricles during contraction. In the clinical setting a rise in afterload, particularly in the failing heart, results in a decrease in cardiac output (Lee & Branch 1997). Table 3.3 lists factors affecting afterload.

Table 3.2 Factors affecting preload

Factors increasing preload:	volume gain, e.g. fluid overload; renal failure; vasoconstriction (may be caused by drugs, e.g. noradrenaline, adrenaline & dopamine (dose related)); heart failure; hypothermia and anxiety; bradycardia
Factors decreasing preload:	volume loss, e.g. haemorrhage, severe vomiting & polyuria; vasodilatation, e.g. anaphylaxis, septicaemia, pyrexia, neurogenic shock & drugs such as nitrates; impeded venous return, e.g. pulmonary embolism, pericardial tamponade; tachycardia (fall in diastolic filling time)

Table 3.3 Factors affecting afterload

Factors that increase afterload:	drugs with vasoconstriction properties, e.g. noradrenaline; cardiogenic shock; atherosclerosis
Factors that decrease afterload:	drugs with vasodilator properties, e.g. nitrates, nitropruside; anaphylaxsis; septicaemia; hyperthermia

Peripheral resistance

Peripheral resistance is the resistance to the flow of blood determined by the tone of the vascular musculature and the diameter of the blood vessels (Mosby 1998).

The smooth muscle in the arterioles is controlled by the vasomotor centre in the medulla. It is in a state of partial contraction caused by continuous sympathetic nerve activity, often referred to as 'sympathetic tone'.

An increase in vasomotor activity causes vasoconstriction of the arterioles resulting in a rise in peripheral resistance. If the cardiac output remains constant the blood pressure will rise. In contrast a decrease in vasomotor activity causes vasodilation and a fall in peripheral resistance. If the cardiac output remains constant the blood pressure will fall. The most significant factors affecting vasomotor activity are listed below.

- *Baroreceptor activity* helps to maintain the blood pressure at a constant level. Baroreceptors are located in the aortic arch, carotid arteries and carotid sinus. Baroreceptor activity inhibits the action of the vasomotor centre: a rise in blood pressure increases, and a fall decreases, baroreceptor activity. When moving from a lying to a standing position, the cardiac output will fall. However baroreceptor activity ensures that the blood pressure remains constant. Following prolonged bed rest this mechanism may be lost and the patient may faint.
- *Carbon dioxide (CO$_2$)*: a rise in blood CO$_2$ levels increases vasomotor activity, whilst a fall suppresses it. In ventilated patients care needs to be taken to avoid over-ventilation as this may lead to a fall in CO$_2$ levels with a corresponding fall in blood pressure.
- *Sensory nerves* can influence vasomotor activity, particularly those which are associated with pain. Mild pain can increase vasomotor activity resulting in a rise in blood pressure, whilst severe pain may decrease vasomotor activity and cause a fall in blood pressure.
- *Respiratory centre*: this lies next to the vasomotor centre; an increase in its activity, particularly on inspiration, will result in an increase in vasomotor activity causing a rise in blood pressure.
- *Oxygen (O$_2$)*: a moderate fall in blood oxygen levels increases vasomotor activity directly and also indirectly via chemoreceptors.
- *Higher centres*: emotional excitement or stress results in a rise in vasomotor activity and a corresponding rise in blood pressure. In some situations inhibition of the vasomotor centre will occur resulting in vasodilation and a fall in blood pressure, for instance, some people faint at the sight of blood.

There are other factors that affect peripheral resistance including:

- *angiotensin*: inadequate renal blood flow leads to the release of the enzyme renin which causes the formation of angiotensin, a powerful vasoconstrictor;
- *blood viscosity*: if the blood viscosity increases, e.g. in polycythaemia peripheral resistance will also rise;
- *stimulation of alpha and beta 2 receptors* (found in the smooth muscle of the arterioles): stimulation of alpha receptors, e.g. by noradrenaline will cause vasoconstriction; stimulation of beta 2 receptors, e.g. by salbutamol will cause vasodilation.

CLASSIFICATION OF CIRCULATORY SHOCK

'Circulatory shock may be defined as a state of cardiovascular dysfunction resulting in a generalised inadequacy of tissue perfusion relative to metabolic requirements. Tissue hypoxia leads to progressive failure of cellular metabolism, eventually resulting in multiple organ dysfunction or death.'

(Skowronski 1997)

Haemodynamic monitoring will assist in the early recognition of shock, where the immediate provision of circulatory support is paramount (Hinds & Watson 1999).

The prognosis of shock will depend on the underlying cause, severity and duration of the shocked state. The patient's age and pre-existing illness are also contributing factors. There are four classifications of shock (Hinds & Watson 1999).

Hypovolaemic shock

Although the heart may be pumping effectively, loss of circulating volume reduces O_2 delivery. Causes include haemorrhaging, burns, severe vomiting and diarrhoea. It can also be a complication of intestinal obstruction.

Cardiogenic shock

Cardiogenic shock follows cardiac pump failure although there is adequate circulatory volume. Causes include myocardial infarction, cardiac arrhythmias and myocarditis.

Haemodynamic readings show low cardiac output, high pulmonary artery wedge pressure, an increase in SVR and a fall in LVSW (Green 1991)

Distributive shock

This arises from abnormality of the peripheral circulation. Causes include sepsis, neurogenic and anaphylaxis. Cardiac output may rise but O_2 uptake is impaired and a relative low volume is present because of increased intravascular space caused by dilation of the systemic vasculature.

Haemodynamic readings appear normal or show an increase in cardiac output, a fall in SVR and low to normal pulmonary artery wedge pressure.

Obstructive shock

This is caused by mechanical obstruction to cardiac filling and therefore cardiac output. Causes include pulmonary embolism, tension pneumothorax and cardiac tamponade.

Haemodynamic readings show a fall in cardiac output, fall in pulmonary artery wedge pressure and a rise in SVR. Pressures of right side of the heart, pulmonary artery and left chambers are equilibreate in diastole, while cardiac output falls, SVR rises and pulmonary artery wedge pressure is variable dependent on the cause of the obstruction.

NON-INVASIVE METHODS OF
HAEMODYNAMIC MONITORING

This section discusses the various non-invasive methods of haemodynamic monitoring. A non-invasive monitoring device is illustrated in Fig. 3.2.

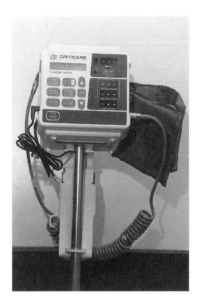

Fig. 3.2 Non-invasive blood pressure monitoring device.

Assessment of pulse and ECG

A rapid, weak, thready pulse is a characteristic sign of shock. A full bounding or throbbing pulse may be indicative of anaemia, heart block, heart failure or the early stages of septic shock. A discrepancy in the volume between central and distal pulses may be caused by a fall in cardiac output (and also cold ambient temperature).

ECG monitoring is an invaluable non-invasive method of continuous monitoring of the heart rate. It can provide the practitioner with an early sign of a fall in cardiac output. The principles of ECG monitoring have been discussed in Chapter 2.

Assessment of cerebral perfusion

Clinical signs of poor cerebral perfusion include a deterioration in conscious level, confusion, agitation and lethargy.

Assessment of skin perfusion

Decreased skin perfusion is often characterised by cool peripheries, skin mottling, pallor, cyanosis and delayed capillary refill (>2 s). The following procedure is suggested for the assessment of capillary refill.

- Explain the procedure to the patient.
- Elevate the extremity, e.g. digit, slightly higher than the level of the heart (this will ensure the assessment of arteriolar capillary and not venous stasis refill).
- Blanch the digit for five seconds and then release. A sluggish (delayed) capillary refill (>2 s) may be caused by circulatory shock, pyrexia or a cold ambient temperature.

Assessment of urine output

Urine output can indirectly provide an indication to cardiac output. In health 25% of the cardiac output perfuses the kidneys. When renal perfusion is adequate, urine output should exceed 0.5 ml/kg per hour (Gomersall & Oh 1997).

A diminished urine output may be caused by a fall in cardiac output and renal perfusion. If diuretics have been administered, e.g. frusemide or dopamine, urine output is not helpful in assessing cardiac output (Duke *et al.* 1994). If the patient is catheterised, ensure that the tube is not blocked or kinked.

Arterial blood pressure measurements

Arterial blood pressure (ABP) is the force exerted by the circulating volume of blood on the walls of the arteries (Mosby 1998). Changes in cardiac output or peripheral resistance can affect the blood pressure. A patient with a low cardiac output can maintain a normal blood pressure by vasoconstriction, whilst a patient who is vasodilated may be hypotensive despite a high cardiac output, e.g. in sepsis.

'The adequacy of blood pressure in an individual patient must always be assessed in relation to their premorbid value'

Table 3.4 Normal intracardiac pressures

Central venous	0 to +8 mmHg (right atrial level)
Right ventricle	0 to +8 mmHg diastolic +15 to + 30 mmHg systolic
Pulmonary capillary wedge pressure	+5 to +15 mmHg
Left atrium	+4 to +12 mmHg
Left ventricle	+4 to + 12 mmHg diastolic +90 to +140 mmHg systolic
Aorta	+90 to +140 mmHg systolic +60 to +90 mmHg diastolic +70 to +105 mmHg mean

Reproduced with kind permission of Routledge from Woodrow 2000

(Hinds & Watson 1996). Table 3.4 provides an indication to 'expected' systolic and diastolic blood pressure measurements. Hypotension can lead to inadequate perfusion of vital organs. Hypertension increases myocardial workload and can precipitate cerebral vascular accidents.

Cardiac output is related to pulse pressure, which is the difference between the systolic and diastolic pressures, usually 30–40 mmHg (Mosby 1998). Following a fall in cardiac output the pulse pressure will narrow, resulting in a thready pulse. In the early stages of septic shock, the cardiac output can rise, resulting in a wide pulse pressure and bounding pulses.

Factors influencing blood pressure measurements

There are numerous factors that can influence blood pressure, e.g. nicotine, anxiety, pain, position of patient, medications, exercise. It is important to ensure a standardised approach is used to minimise the impact of extraneous variables on blood pressure (Torrance & Semple 1997a, b, c).

Although the blood pressure reading in the left arm is generally a more accurate reflection of arterial blood pressure

(Torrance & Semple 1997a, b, c), blood pressure measurement should be recorded in the arm with the highest reading (O'Brien *et al.* 1995). Wide discrepancies between right and left arm blood pressure measurements may be indicative of an aortic aneurysm.

Factors affecting accuracy of blood pressure measurements

The accuracy of blood pressure measurement may be affected by the following factors.

- *Cuff width*: if this is too narrow the blood pressure reading will be falsely high while if too wide it will be falsely low (Gomersall & Oh 1997). The European Standard recommends that the width of the bladder should be 40%, and the length 80–100%, of the limb circumference (CEN 1995).
- *Position of the arm*: the arm should be supported in a horizontal position at the level of the heart. Incorrect positioning during the procedure can lead to errors of as much as 10% (O'Brien *et al.* 1995).

Complications

Complications associated with non-invasive blood pressure devices include limb oedema, friction blisters and ulnar nerve palsy if the cuff is placed too low on the upper arm (Gomersall & Oh 1997). If the patient is being thrombylised, e.g. following myocardial infarction, over inflation or frequent inflations could cause excessive bruising (Smith 2000).

GENERAL PRINCIPLES OF MONITORING WITH TRANSDUCERS

Transducers enable the pressure readings from invasive monitoring of the patient to be displayed on a monitor. To maintain patency of the cannula and tubing and prevent backflow of blood, a bag of normal saline should be connected to the transducer tubing and kept under continuous pressure of

300 mmHg (i.e. > arterial pressure), thus facilitating a continuous flush at 3 ml per hour.

Best practice – monitoring with transducers

Check flush bag each shift – if it runs too low the line will clot off

If flat trace check for breaks in the circuit and air – rectify safely and flush line

If trace remains flat withdraw blood while manipulating limb

Always check the patient – asystole causes a flat trace

Ensuring accuracy
The following precautions will help to ensure accuracy of measurements.

- Keep the transducer level with the zero reference point, usually the mid-axilla. Always use the same reference point in order to ensure meaningful comparison.
- Limit the use of three way taps.
- Remove any air bubbles from the system.
- Calibrate the transducer to atmospheric pressure prior to and regularly during use. This should be undertaken following the manufacturer's recommendations and is typically as follows:
  (1) switch the three way tap in the tubing open to air (atmospheric pressure) and off to the patient;
  (2) press the zero button on the monitor and observe for 0 to be displayed;
  (3) switch the three way tap off to air and open to the patient;
  (4) ensure that the transducer is at the zero reference point and observe for the pressure trace on the monitor.

Principles of arterial pressure monitoring
Indications for insertion of an arterial line include the requirement for continuous monitoring of arterial blood pressure

required, e.g. if patient is on inotropic and/vasoactive drugs and frequent arterial blood sampling, e.g. blood gas and acid base analysis.

Best practice – monitoring an arterial line

Ensure arterial line is clearly labelled 'arterial'

Limb should be exposed and constantly observed for signs of a decrease in perfusion and disconnection of the cannula

Use transparent dressing so site can be monitored for signs of infection

Ensure monitor alarms are set following local protocols

If flat trace observed, once asystole excluded, identify and rectify cause of problem

---

Common insertion sites

The radial artery (alternative sites include the brachial, dorsalis pedis and femoral arteries) is usually the site of choice; advantages include:

- superficial position;
- readily accessible;
- easy to monitor and observe;
- easy to apply pressure in the event of bleeding;
- minimal restriction to patient movement;
- adequate collateral circulation is normally present (Hinds & Watson 1999).

The arterial waveform

The arterial waveform reflects the pressure generated in the arteries following ventricular contraction. Figure 3.3 depicts a typical arterial waveform and its configuration can be described as follows.

- *Anacrotic notch*: peak systolic pressure.
- *Peak systolic pressure*: this reflects maximum left ventricular systolic pressure.

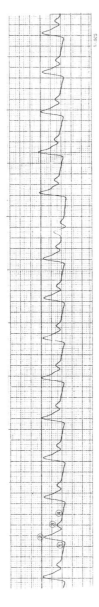

Fig. 3.3 Arterial waveform. 1. anacrotic notch; 2. peak systolic pressure; 3. dicrotic notch, and 4. diastolic pressure.

- *Dicrotic notch*: reflects aortic valve closure. It is notably elevated in patients with increased peripheral resistance and decreased cardiac output.
- *Diastolic pressure*: reflects the degree of vasoconstriction in the arterial system.

Complications of arterial line insertion

Nurses need to be constantly alert to the possible complications of arterial line insertion. These include exanguination, ischaemia distal to the cannula and tissue necrosis, inadvertent administration of drugs into the artery, air embolus and thrombosis.

Table 3.5 summarises the problems associated with arterial lines.

Monitoring priorities of a patient with an arterial line

The following measures should always be observed when a patient with an arterial line is being monitored.

- Ensure the tubing and cannula are secured.
- Clearly label the tubing 'arterial' to help prevent accidental arterial injection of drugs (Mallett & Dougherty 2000).
- Use a transparent dressing so that any dislodgement or disconnection will be immediately recognised.
- Ensure that the limb is visible at all times to monitor perfusion and closed circuit.
- Regularly assess tissue perfusion distal to the cannula site. Thrombosis or the development of an adjacent haematoma could jeopardise arterial blood flow. If signs of poor tissue perfusion are present, e.g. if the limb becomes white, cold or painful, inform medical staff immediately – the line will need to be removed.
- Regularly assess the site for signs of infection. Replace dressing if soiled.
- Maintain a bag of 0.9% normal saline at a pressure of 300 mgHg to help maintain patency and change it following locally agreed protocols.

Table 3.5 Summary of potential problems associated with an arterial cannula

Problem	Cause	Action
'Damped' trace (Fig. 3.4) leading to underestimated BP (blunt pressure peak, loss of dicrotic notch)	Loss of pressure or no fluid in the infusion pressure bag.	Inflate pressure bag to 300 mmHg. Check there is sufficient flushing fluid.
	Thrombus/fibrin formation at tip of catheter.	Withdraw blood and then flush catheter.
	Air in tubing or transducer	Disconnect tubing from catheter and flush through to expel air before reconnecting. If necessary, change transducer.
	Too many 3-way taps in the circuit.	Remove excess taps.
	Long length of tubing between catheter and transducer.	Shorten tubing.
	Poor position of limb, tip of catheter against vessel wall, kinked tubing.	Manipulate catheter and/or limb to achieve a better trace.
No arterial waveform (straight line)	Taps turned off to patient or transducer.	Check taps are on to patient and transducer.
	Disconnection of catheter.	Check catheter site – reconnect immediately.
	Disconnection of transducer cable to monitor.	Check connections – reconnect .
	Poor catheter position (tip against vessel wall).	Manipulate position, flush catheter.
	Asystole.	Institute CPR.
Backflow of blood from catheter towards transducer	Loose tap connection within the circuit.	Check all connections are secure.
	Flush bag pressure too low (below patient's BP).	Inflate bag to 300 mmHg pressure.

- Ensure all connections are secure. Exsanguination through a 18 FG cannula can lead to blood loss of 500 ml per minute (Gomersall & Oh 1997). Extra vigilance is required if the femoral artery has been used because the site will be covered up. If the cannula is transduced alarms should be appropriately set to alert the nurse to any disruption in the pressures indicating disconnection.
- Only competent practitioners should undertake arterial blood sampling.
- Use minimum amount of 'taps' to reduce the risk of infection, leakage and inadvertent drug administration.

Trouble shooting – flat arterial trace

If a flat arterial trace is observed on the monitor check the:

- patient is not in asystole
- circuit connections
- circuit for air bubbles and safely remove if present
- tubing in the circuit is not kinked
- flush bag has adequate fluid and a sufficient pressure is being maintained
- proximal joint as the cannula may be kinked or compressed against the vessel wall – repositioning the joint may be necessary
- patency of the arterial cannula by withdrawing blood
- patient's blood pressure manually

Once the problem has been rectified flush and re-zero line

PRINCIPLES OF CENTRAL VENOUS PRESSURE MONITORING

Central venous pressure (CVP) reflects right atrial filling pressure or preload. The normal CVP is 0–8 mmHg (Woodrow 2000). A low CVP reading usually indicates hypovolaemia while a high CVP reading has a number of causes including hypervolaemia, cardiac failure and pulmonary embolism.

Indications for CVP lines

Central venous pressure monitoring is used in a variety of procedures:

- fluid resuscitation;
- parenteral feeding;
- measurement of central venous pressure;
- poor venous access;
- administration of irritant drugs.

The usual sites for insertion of CVP lines are internal jugular (right and left) and subclavian (right or left). The latter is often the preferred site. Although the subclavian has more recognisable landmarks to aid the clinician there are fewer risks associated with the internal jugular.

The femoral vein is sometimes used but generally only as a last resort because of the increased risk of colonisation (Gil *et al.* 1989 and Goetz *et al.* 1998). Central venous catheters can be single, triple, quadruple or quintuple lumened. Strict asepsis must be adhered to on insertion and following management as microorganisms that colonise catheter hubs and the skin adjacent to the insertion site are the source of most catheter related blood stream infections (Department of Health 2001).

There is recent evidence to suggest that microbial impregnated central venous catheters used short-term (<7 days) reduce the risk of catheter related blood stream infections (Mermel 2000), although these have only been recently available in the UK.

Central venous pressure (CVP) monitoring can be helpful in the assessment of cardiac function, circulating blood volume, vascular tone and the patient's response to treatment. However CVP can be influenced by a number of factors and should therefore be interpreted in combination with other systemic measurements. An isolated CVP measurement can be misleading; a trend is of more value.

To help ensure validity of the measurements and accuracy of their interpretation, the patient's position should be constant (supine if possible) and the same point of reference (mid-axilla) should be used for each reading.

Methods of CVP monitoring

There are two methods of CVP monitoring:

- *manometer system*: enables intermittent readings and is less accurate than the transducer system;
- *transducer system*: enables continuous readings which are displayed on a monitor.

Procedure for CVP measurement using a manometer

(1) Explain the procedure to the patient.

(2) Ensure patency of the central venous catheter prior to the procedure – this can normally be ascertained by checking that the flush is working or by drawing blood back.

(3) Position the patient supine, if possible. The same position should be used for each measurement to help ensure the trend of readings is accurate.

(4) Align the manometer arm with the mid-axilla, ensuring that the 'bubble' is in between the lines on the spirit level. The reading on the manometer scale at this level should be zero (the baseline of the manometer scale is now level with the right atrium). Use the same point of reference for each measurement.

(5) Turn the three way tap off to the patient and on to the manometer. Check the fluid source ensuring it is the correct solution to use (usually normal saline) and does not contain drugs.

(6) Switch on the fluid source and slowly fill up the manometer tubing to above the expected reading. Care should be taken to ensure the manometer tubing fills up slowly. This will help avoid air bubbles which can lead to an inaccurate reading and prevent over-filling of, and spillage from, the manometer which is an infection risk (Mallett & Dougherty 2000).

(7) Turn the three way tap 'off' to the fluid source and 'on' to the patient. The fluid level in the manometer tubing

should fall rapidly. This will allow fluid from the manometer to enter the right atrium.

(8) Once the fluid level stops falling (it should be oscillating with the patient's respirations) the reading can then be taken using the lower reading.

(9) Turn the three way tap off to the patient (reconnect infusion fluids if appropriate).

(10) Document the reading and report any changes or abnormalities.

Procedure for CVP measurement using a transducer

(1) Explain the procedure to the patient.

(2) Ensure patency of the central venous catheter prior to the procedure.

(3) Position the patient, supine if possible. The same position should be used for each measurement.

(4) Calibrate (zero) the monitor following the manufacturer's recommendations – this usually involves opening the system to the atmosphere (off to the patient, open to air) and pressing a 'zero' button on the monitor; once zero is displayed the monitor has been calibrated). Zeroing a CVP removes extraneous pressure (Henderson 1997).

(5) Observe the CVP trace on the monitor. The waveform on the monitor should be slightly undulating in nature (Fig. 3.5), reflecting changes in right atrial pressure during the cardiac cycle.

(6) Document the reading and report any changes and abnormalities (also calculate mean pressure reading).

The CVP waveform

The CVP waveform reflects changes in right atrial pressure during the cardiac cycle. Figure 3.5 depicts a typical CVP waveform and its configuration can be described as follows.

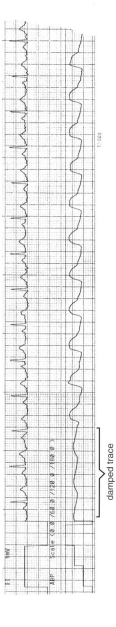

Fig. 3.4 Damped arterial trace

- *A wave: right atrial contraction (P wave on the ECG)*. If the A wave is elevated the patient may have right ventricular failure or tricuspid stenosis.
- *C wave: tricuspid valve closure (follows QRS complex on the ECG)*. The distance from A–C should correlate with the P–R interval on the ECG.
- *V wave: pressure generated to the right atrium during ventricular contraction, despite the tricuspid valve being closed (latter part of the T wave on the ECG)*. If the V wave is elevated the patient may have tricuspid valve disease.

Tunnelling of central venous catheters under the skin can prevent the risk of catheter related blood stream infection (Randolph *et al.* 1998), although this has not been demonstrated with the femoral site (Timsit *et al.* 1996).

Normal CVP measurements

Central venous pressure monitoring should normally show measurements as follows.

Mid axilla: 5–10 cm water (Henderson 1997)

or 0–8 mmHg (Woodrow 2000)

NB: an isolated CVP reading is of limited value; a trend of readings is much more significant and should be viewed in conjunction with other parameters, e.g. BP and urine output.

Trouble shooting

Hinds and Watson (1996) identified the following pitfalls with CVP monitoring.

- *Occluded catheter*: this will result in a persistent high reading with a dampened trace. Ensure that the catheter is patent.
- *Incorrect calibration*: if a transducer and oscilloscope is used, the system should be calibrated following the manufacturer's recommendations.
- *Inconsistent procedure for measurements*: ensure consistent

procedure (identical patient position and point of reference) for serial CVP measurements.

- *Infusion(s) in progress*: a falsely high CVP measurement will result if infusion(s) continue to be administered through the CVP catheter during the procedure. In addition if the infusion fluid contains vasoactive drugs, the resultant 'flush' can cause a sudden period of cardiac instability. Infusion(s) should be temporarily switched off while CVP measurement is undertaken (ideally all infusions should be administered through other catheters).

- *Catheter tip in the right ventricle*: this will result in an unexpected high pressure reading. If the patient is transduced the presenting waveform will confirm suspicions.

- *Respiratory oscillations*: measurements should be taken at end-expiration, especially if the patient is in respiratory distress or is being ventilated, as the central venous pressure will be artificially higher because of positive intrathoracic pressure.

Complications following CVP line insertion

Nurses should be alert to the possibility of complications following CVP line insertion:

- malposition of the catheter (Czepizak *et al*. 1995) (Fig. 3.6);
- haematoma (Gilbert *et al*. 1995);
- arterial puncture (Robinson *et al*. 1995);
- pneumothorax (Sznajder *et al*. 1986);
- haemorrhage;
- sepsis;
- air emboli: although < 20 ml of air rarely causes problems (Hudak *et al*. 1998) larger volumes of air could cause a pulmonary embolism and cardiac arrest;
- thrombosis: serious thrombosis occurs following 4–35% of central line insertion (Kaye & Smth 1988);
- ventricular perforation;
- cardiac arrhythmias.

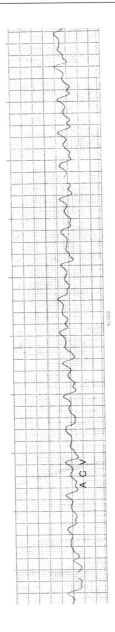

Fig. 3.5 CVP trace. A, C and V waves.

Management of a patient with a CVP line

The precautions listed below should always be observed.

- Monitor the patient for signs of complications.
- Label CVP lines with drugs/fluids, etc. being infused in order to minimise the risk of accidental bolus injection.
- If not in use, flush the cannula regularly to help prevent thrombosis. A 500 ml bag of 0.9% normal saline should be maintained at a pressure of 150 mmHg and changed on a daily basis following locally agreed protocols. As an alternative use regular bolus injections of normal saline.
- Ensure all connections are secure to prevent exsanguination, introduction of infection and air emboli.
- Observe the insertion site frequently for signs of infection. Transparent dressings should be used to permit continuous monitoring of the site. The incidence of CVP line related infection ranges from 4%-18%. If infection of the CVP line is suspected blood cultures should be taken following removal of the line. The catheter tip should be sent for MC & S. The length of the indwelling catheter should be recorded and regularly monitored. The dressing should be changed as required, ensuring strict aseptic technique.
- Although the routine replacement of CVP lines is widespread in the UK (Cyna *et al.* 1998), this is not recommended as such practice is associated with a higher incidence of morbidity and mortality in critically ill patients. In addition replacing a CVP line is not only expensive and traumatic for the patient, but there is also an added risk of introducing an infection (Clemence *et al.* 1995). CVP lines should therefore only be removed when clinically indicated (O'Leary & Bihari 1998).
- Be alert to possible complications identified above.

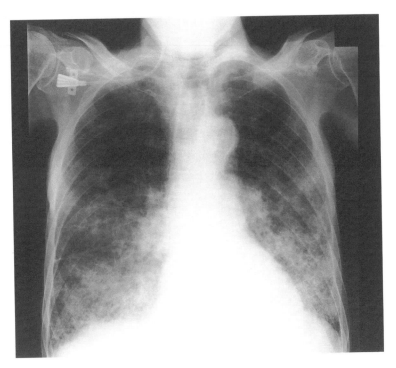

Fig. 3.6 Malposition of the CVP catheter – patient with known COPD and basal pulmonary fibrosis. The right subclavian line tip is pointing cranially with the tip in the internal jugular vein. (We are grateful to Louise Holland, Consultant Radiologist at the Manor Hospital Walsall for her assistance.)

PRINCIPLES OF PULMONARY ARTERY PRESSURE MONITORING

Pulmonary artery catheter

Since it was first described by Swan and Ganz in the 1970s, the pulmonary artery (PA) catheter which is also known as a multi lumen directional flow catheter (Fig. 3.7) has been widely used for the diagnosis and treatment of critically ill patients.

It can be used to evaluate cardiac function and to detect

problems in the pulmonary vasculature and enables the clinician to optimise cardiac output and delivery of oxygen whilst minimising the risk of pulmonary oedema; it also allows the rational use of vasoactive and inotropic drugs (Hinds & Watson 1999). Quite often it provides unexpected haemodynamic information, resulting in changes in treatment (Mimoz *et al.* 1994).

The use of the PA catheter is not without risk. Although common in the ITU environment, there is no evidence that its use improves survival rates (Eidelman *et al.* 1994); in fact there are reports that it may increase mortality rates. Therefore the use of PA catheters should be limited to experienced, well trained clinicians familiar with the interpretation of data derived from the catheter who are able to adjust treatment based on the results obtained.

There are many recommendations for the most appropriate use of PA catheters; however, there is no consensus agreement on how the patient's treatment should be adjusted based on the collected data (Swan & Ganz 1974; European Society of Intensive Care Medicine 1991).

Indications

Use of PA pressure is indicated for:

- assessment of circulatory volume and fluid management in impaired right or left ventricular function or pulmonary hypertension;
- cardiac output measurements;
- mixed venous saturation measurements;
- diagnosis of ventricular septal defect.

Gomersall & Oh 1997

Waveform as pulmonary artery catheter passes from the vena cava to the pulmonary artery

Figure 3.8 depicts the pressure traces seen as a pulmonary artery catheter passes from the vena cava to the pulmonary artery. Pulmonary vasculature is more compliant than the

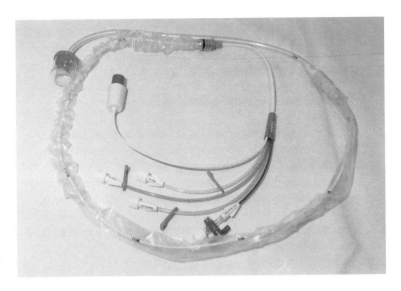

Fig. 3.7 Pulmonary artery catheter.

systemic vessels, consequently pulmonary pressures are lower (Table 3.5) (Woodrow 2000). Pulmonary hypertension is common in ICU patients, e.g. those with ARDS. If the pulmonary artery pressure is low despite a high CVP this is indicative of right sided heart failure (Woodrow 2000).

Pressures

Using a pulmonary catheter it is possible to measure the pressures in the right atrium (RA), right ventricle (RV) and pulmonary artery (PA)(see Table 3.5):

- RA pressure: during ventricular filling is 0–8 mmHg;
- RV pressure: end diastolic pressure is 0–8 mmHg, systolic pressure 15–30 mmHg;
- PA pressure: diastolic 5–15 mmHg, systolic 15–30 mmHg.

A high diastolic pressure indicates right heart failure, pulmonary hypertension or tamponade. High PA pressure indicates LVF or pulmonary hypertension, low PA pressure is suggestive of hypovolaemia.

Cardiac index (CI) is cardiac output indexed to individual body surface area. Normal is between 2.4 and $41/min/m^2$. These readings may never be completely precise as it is very difficult to weigh and measure a very sick patient accurately. The relevance however, is in the trend of results that the Swan Ganz catheter facilitates and the response to treatment administered.

Pulmonary artery wedge pressure (PAWP)

If the balloon is inflated in the branch of the pulmonary artery, the pressure at the tip of the catheter will reflect the pressure distal to it, i.e. left atrial and ventricular pressure which is in direct correlation to preload.

Procedure

(1) Explain the procedure to the patient.
(2) Watching the monitor at the same time, slowly inflate the balloon until the characteristic flattened waveform is identified (Fig. 3.8). The balloon is now 'wedged', i.e. it is occluding the blood flow in the vessel.
(3) Stop inflating the balloon and allow the trace to run for three respiratory cycles (very important).
(4) Freeze the monitor screen and deflate the balloon rapidly.
(5) Ascertain the wedge pressure by aligning the cursor control on the monitor to the correct position on the waveform (end expiration).
(6) Unfreeze the monitor screen and ensure the pulmonary artery waveform is present.

Precautions

Care should be taken to observe the following precautions.

• Do not leave the balloon inflated for longer than three respiratory cycles (15 s).

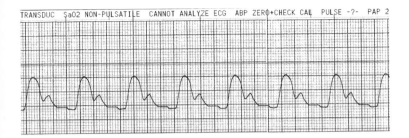

Fig. 3.8 Pressure traces seen as the pulmonary artery catheter passes from the vena cava to the pulmonary artery.

- Do not inflate more that 1.5 ml of air into the balloon.
- Do not flush the catheter if the balloon is inflated.
- If the trace rises sharply during balloon inflation, then the catheter is over-wedged.

Limitations
Pulmonary artery wedge pressure does not accurately reflect left atrial and ventricular pressure in:

- pulmonary venous obstruction;
- mitral stenosis;
- left atrial myxoma (very rare).

Normal wedge range is 5–15 mmHg (Woodrow 2000) and should correlate with the pulmonary artery diastolic pressure – a high reading may signify LVF, mitral insufficiency or fluid overload whereas a low reading may signify hypovolaemia.

Systemic vascular resistance (SVR) is the measurement of afterload and a critical measurement in the diagnosis and treatment of sepsis. Normal is 900–1400 dynes/s/cm-5. SVRI is indexed to body surface area calculated from weight and height.

Complications
Complications resulting following PA catheter use include:

- cardiac arrhythmias;
- thrombosis;
- pulmonary infarction;
- rupture of the pulmonary artery – often associated with balloon inflation during measuring the wedge pressure (Leeper 1995);
- myocardial perforation (Daily & Schroeder 1989);
- knotting of the catheter (Tan *et al*. 1997).

CARDIAC OUTPUT STUDIES

Thermodilution

Thermodilution is the most popular method for measuring cardiac output. It is important that the readings are taken following interventions, e.g. titration of vasoactive drugs or fluid bolus. It involves a rapid injection of a measured amount of cold fluid (usually 5–10 ml of 5% dextrose) into the right atrium through the proximal lumen of the PA catheter. Its dilution by the blood is calculated by serial changes in PA temperature. The cardiac output is calculated on the basis of the temperature change: the rise in solution temperature is inversely related to the functioning of the heart.

Indications

Thermodilution is indicated in clinical situations where the assessment of volaemic status and cardiac output along with haemodynamic variables will help in the diagnosis and management. For example:

- management and diagnosis of all forms of shock;
- impaired right or left ventricular function as seen in cardiac failure;
- measurement of cardiac output;
- measurement of mixed venous saturation;
- diagnosis of ventricular septal defect.

Procedure

(1) Explain the procedure to the patient.

(2) Draw up the injection fluid.

(3) Ensure that the injection fluid is lower than body temperature.

(4) Flush the proximal port with the injection fluid; the injection fluid displayed on the monitor should be within the accepted range for the monitoring system.

(5) Ensure that the monitor is ready.

(6) Press the start button on the monitor and inject 5–10 ml smoothly within four seconds (do not hold the syringe barrel, as this could warm the injection fluid). Approximately 15 seconds later, the cardiac output measurement will be displayed on the monitor. After about 45 seconds, the monitor will display 'ready' again.

(7) Press the start button again and repeat the above procedure. At least three measurements should be made and an average worked out.

Troubleshooting

The following problems are associated with thermodilution cardiac output measurements (Adam & Osborne 1997).

- *Difficulty injecting the solution*: the tube may be kinked or occluded or the catheter tip may be positioned against the vessel wall. Unkink, reposition or replace catheter as necessary.

- *Blood temperature not displayed*: the thermistor may be faulty or may have a fibrin growth attached. Replace the catheter if necessary.

- *Injection fluid temperature not displayed*: replace the faulty temperature probe.

- *Major discrepancies in serial measurements*: possible causes include poor injection technique, cardiac arrhythmias (causing varying stroke volumes), and vascular disease causing turbulent blood and patient movement. Adhere to procedure described above, do not inject during arrhythmic episodes and limit patient movement during injection.

- *Inappropriately high cardiac output measurements*: possible causes include incorrect injection fluid volume (usually too little or leaking connection), injection fluid temperature too low, poor injection technique and computer error. Adhere to the procedure described above and if indicated check the computer.
- *Inappropriately low cardiac output measurements*: possible causes include incorrect injection fluid volume (usually too much), injection fluid temperature too high, start button on the monitor pressed after starting the injection, computer error, prolonged injection time and concomitant fluid infusion through the distal lumen. Adhere to the procedure described above and if indicated check the computer.

Mixed venous oxygen saturation

Mixed venous oxygen saturation (SVO_2) represents the amount of oxygen, which remains after perfusion of the capillary beds and is an indicator of the balance between oxygen delivery and oxygen consumption (Takala 1997).

SVO_2 measurements, which can be used as a guide to tissue perfusion, are directly proportional to cardiac output, haemoglobin and oxygen saturation levels and inversely with the metabolic rate (Gomersall & Oh 1997).

- SVO_2 75%: normal.
- $SVO_2 \leq 75\%$: low. If the oxygen delivery drops or if tissue oxygen demand rises this can lead to a low measurement. If $SVO_2 < 30\%$ then oxygen delivery is insufficient to meet the oxygen needs of the tissues.
- $SVO_2 \geq 75\%$: high, can be difficult to interpret. Causes include sepsis, hypothermia, cyanide poisoning, left to right cardiac shunts (Gomersall & Oh 1997).

Methods for SVO_2 measurements

SVO_2 measurement may be performed in two ways:

- *intermittent* blood sampling from the distal PA catheter or *continuously* through a fibreoptic PA catheter;
- a co-oximeter is also required because blood gas machines are unable to calculate lower SVO_2

Non-invasive methods of measuring cardiac output

Because of the invasive nature of Swan Ganz catheters and their associated complications, it is always preferable to use non-invasive methods if available to measure cardiac function.

Cardiac output monitor

This monitor (Fig. 3.9) calculates cardiac output by the use of the Fick principle based upon the partial re-breathing of CO_2. This system can only be used on a ventilated patient and analyses CO_2 production and thereby calculates cardiac output.

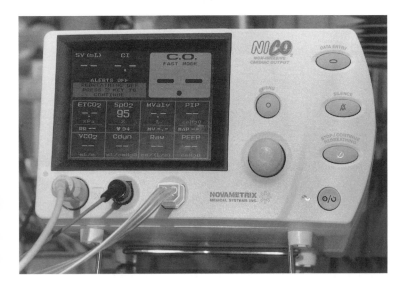

Fig. 3.9 Non-invasive cardiac output monitor.

Transoesophageal Doppler

This involves placing a Doppler inside the oesophagus and echo imaging of blood flow turbulence through the aorta is demonstrated. It is accurate within 2.9% of thermodilution cardiac output studies (Tibby *et al*. 1997) and the majority of measurements are underestimates (Hinds & Watson 1999). It is only suitable for sedated or ventilated patients and can cause oesophageal trauma (Valtier *et al*. 1998).

SCENARIOS

Scenario 1

Mrs Cook, a 45-year-old with known gall stones, was admitted with right upper quadrant pain, pyrexia and malaise. She was diagnosed with ascending cholangitis and commenced on cefotaxime 2 g IV TDS and metronidazole 500 mg IV TDS.

On day two of admission she developed a BP of 80/60, HR 120 and resps 35/min. She was warm to the touch with warm peripheries. She was transferred to ICU as her conscious level deteriorated. Septic shock was suspected and urgent surgical review requested.

A Swan Ganz catheter was inserted and the following readings were obtained:

PAOP 12 mmHg

CO 7.0 l/min

SVR slightly low

CVP 8 mmHg

LVSW high normal

What do these results show?

Septic shock was confirmed and fluid resuscitation together with noradrenaline started. Antibiotics were continued and surgical review sought, as identification of the sepsis is paramount.

Scenario 2

Mr Smith, a 54-year-old man, was admitted with an acute myocardial infarction. His observations were within normal limits and he was warm and well perfused. He suddenly developed a broad complex tachycardia, rate 180 per minute. He is conscious, what would you do?

The patient is conscious therefore he must have a pulse (if he was pulseless, CPR and rapid defibrillation would be required). If not already, administer oxygen, secure IV access and establish whether the patient is haemodynamically compromised. Are there any adverse signs? (e.g. systolic blood pressure < 90 mmHg, chest pain, heart failure, rapid rate > 150 (Resuscitation Council UK 2000)).

On examination Mr Smith's pulse was week, rapid (180 per minute) and thready. His blood pressure has fallen to 70 mmHg systolic, he is cold, pale and clammy and his conscious level is deteriorating. What would you do?

He is severely haemodynamically compromised and requires urgent treatment, e.g. cardioversion. If the patient had not been compromised, drugs, e.g. amiodarone or lidocaine would have probably been the first choice of treatment. Any electrolyte imbalance would also need to be treated.

CONCLUSION

Haemodynamic monitoring is central to the care of a critically ill patient. It helps to establish a precise diagnosis, determine appropriate therapy and monitor the response to that therapy. In particular the various methods of haemodynamic monitoring can assist in the early recognition of shock. It is always preferable to utilise the least invasive, yet accurate technique available to reduce the risk of complications for the patient.

Users of monitoring devices must be familiar with the operation of and how to trouble shoot, to minimise the risk of erroneous results.

REFERENCES

Adam, S.K. & Osborne, S. (1997) *Critical Care Nursing: Science and Practice*. Oxford University Press.

CEN European Committee for Standardisation (1995) *EN 1060-1 Non-invasive sphygmomanometers: general requirements*. British Standards Institution, London.

Clemence, M., Walker, D. & Forr, B. (1995) Central venous catheter practices: results of a survey. *American Journal of Infection Control* **23** (1), 5–12.

Cyna, A.M., Hovenden, J.L., Lehmann, A. *et al.* (1998) Routine replacement of central venous catheters: telephone survey of intensive care units in mainland Britain. *British Medical Journal* **316**, 1944–1945.

Czepizak, C.A., O'Callaghan, J.M. & Venus, B. (1995) Evaluation of formulas for optimal positioning of central venous catheters. *Chest* **107**, 1662–1664.

Daily, E.K. & Schroeder, J.S. (1989) *Techniques in Bedside Hemodynamic Monitoring*, 4th edn. C.V. Mosby, London.

Department of Health (2001) Guidelines for preventing infections associated with the insertion and maintenance of central venous catheters. *Journal of Hospital Infection 47 (supplement)* S47–S67

Duke, G.J., Briedis, J.H. & Weaver, R.A. (1994) Renal support in critically ill patients: low dose dopamine or low dose dobutamine? *Critical Care Medicine* **22**, 1919–1925.

Eidelman, L.A., Pizov, R. & Sprung, C.L. (1994) Pulmonary artery catheterisation – at the crossroads? *Critical Care Medicine* **22**, 543–545.

Elliott, T.S.J., Faroqui, M.H., Moss, H.A. *et al.* (1997) *A Guide to the Care and Maintenance of Central Venous Catheters in Adults*. Ohmeda, Hatfield.

European Society of Intensive Care Medicine Expert Panel (1991) The use of the pulmonary artery catheter. *Intensive Care Medicine* **17**, 1–8.

Gil, R., Kruse, J., Thrill-Baharozian, M. & Carolson, R. (1989) Triple versus single lumen central venous catheters: a prospective study in a critically ill population. *Archives of Internal Medicine* **149**, 1139–1143.

Gilbert, T.B., Seneff, M.G. & Becker, R.B. (1995) Facilitation of internal jugular venous cannulation using an audio-guided Doppler ultrasound vascular access device: results from a prospective, dual-center, randomized, cross-over clinical study. *Critical Care Medicine* **23**, 56–65.

Goetz, A., Wagener, M., Miller, J. & Muder, R. (1998) Risk of infection due to central venous catheters: effect of site of placement and catheter type. *Infection Control and Hospital Epidemiology* **19** (11), 842–845.

Gomersall, C. & Oh, T. (1997) Haemodynamic monitoring. In: T. Oh, ed. *Intensive Care Manual*, 4th edn. Butterworth Heinemann, Oxford.

Green, J.H. (1991) *An Introduction to Human Physiology.* Oxford Medical Publications, Oxford.

Henderson, N. (1997) Central venous lines. *Nursing Standard* **11** (42), 49–56.

Hinds, C.J. & Watson, D. (1996) *Intensive Care, a concise textbook* 2nd edn. W.B. Saunders, London.

Hinds, C.J. & Watson, D. (1999) ABC of intensive care: circulatory support. *British Medical Journal* **318**, 1749–1752.

Hudak, C.M., Gallo, B.M. & Morton, P.G. (1998) *Critical Care Nursing: a holistic approach*, 7th edn. Lippincott, New York.

Kaye, C. & Smith, D. (1988) Complications of central venous catheter-isation. *British Medical Journal* **297** (6648), 572–573.

Lee, R. & Branch, J. (1997) Postoperative cardiac intensive care. In: T. Oh ed., *Intensive Care Manual* 4th edn. Butterworth-Heinemann, Oxford.

Leeper, B. (1995) Ask the experts. *Critical Care Nurse* **15**, 82–83.

Mallett, J. & Dougherty, L. (2000) eds *The Royal Marsden Hospital Manual of Clinical Nursing Procedures*. Blackwell Science, Oxford.

Mermel, L. (2000) Prevention of intravascular catheter-related infection. *Annals of Internal Medicine* **32** (5), 391–402.

Mimoz, O., Rauss, A., Rekik, N. *et al.* (1994) Pulmonary artery catheter-isation in critically ill patients: a prospective analysis of outcome changes in therapy. *Critical Care Medicine* **22**, 573–579.

Mosby Publishers (1998) Mosby's Medical, *Nursing and Allied Health Dictionary*, 5th edn. Mosby, London.

O'Brien, E., Beevers, D. & Marshall, H. (1995) *ABC of Hypertension*. BMJ Books, London.

O'Leary, M. & Bihari, D. (1998) Central venous catheters – time for change? *British Medical Journal* **316**, 1918–1919.

Randolph, A., Cook, D., Gonzales, C. & Brun-Buisson, C. (1998) Tunnelling short term central venous catheters to prevent catheter related infection: a meta analysis of randomised controlled trials *Critical Care Medicine* **26** (8), 1452–1457.

Resuscitation Council UK (2000) *Advanced Life Support Manual*, 4th edn. Resuscitation Council UK, London.

Robinson, J.F., Robinson, W.A., Cohn, H. *et al*. (1995) Perforation of the great vessels during central venous line placement. *Archives of Internal Medicine* **155**, 1225–1228.

Skowronski, G. (1997) Circulator shock. In: T. Oh ed., *Intensive Care Manual* 4th edn. Butterworth-Heinemann, Oxford.

Smith, G. (2000) Devices for blood pressure measurement. *Professional Nurse* **15** (5), 337–340.

Soni, N. & Welch, J. (1996) *Invasive Haemodynamic Monitoring*. Ohmeda, Hatfield.

Starling, E.H. (1918) The Law of the Heart. Linacre Lecture, London.

Swan, H.J.C. & Ganz, W. (1974) Guidelines for use of balloon-tipped catheters. *American Journal of Cardiology* **34**, 119–120.

Sznajder, J.I. *et al*. (1986) Central vein catheterisation: failure and complication rates by three percutaneous approaches. *Archives of Internal Medicine* **146**, 259-261.

Takala, J. (1997) Monitoring oxygenation. In: T. Oh, ed. *Intensive Care Manual*, 4th edn. Butterworth Heinemann, Oxford.

Tan, C. *et al*. (1997) A technique to remove knotted pulmonary artery catheters. *Anaesthesia and Intensive Care* **25** (2), 160–162.

Tibby, S., Brock, G., Marsh, M. *et al*. (1997) Haemodynamic monitoring in critically ill children. *Care of the Critically Ill* **13** (3), 86–89.

Timsit, J., Sebille, V., Farkas, J. *et al*. (1996) Effect of tunnelling on internal jugular catheter related sepsis in critically ill patients: a prospective randomized multi-center study. *Journal of the American Medical Association* **276**, 1416–1420.

Torrance, C. & Elley, K. (1997) Respiration, technique and observation 1. *Nursing Times* **93** (43), suppl. 1–2.

Torrance, C. & Semple, M. (1997a) Blood pressure measurement. *Nursing Times* **93** (38), suppl. 1–2.

Torrance, C. & Semple, M. (1997b) Blood pressure measurement. *Nursing Times* **93** (39), suppl. 1–2.

Torrance, C. & Semple, M. (1997c) Blood pressure measurement. *Nursing Times* **93** (40), suppl. 1–2.

Valtier, B., Cholley, B., Belot, J-P. *et al*. (1998) Non-invasive monitoring of cardiac output in critically ill patients using transoesophageal doppler. *American Journal of Respiratory and Critical Care Medicine* **158** (1), 77–83.

Woodrow, P. (2000) *Intensive Care Nursing, A. Framework for Practice*. Routledge, London.

4 | Monitoring Neurological Function

INTRODUCTION

Changes in neurological function can be rapid and dramatic or subtle developing over a period of minutes, hours, days or even longer (Aucken & Crawford 1998). In patients with a head injury or other cerebral insult, monitoring neurological function is essential in order to recognise and treat complications promptly and improve prognosis (Hinds & Watson 1996). It can also provide an indication to the function of other systems, e.g. in renal failure confusion could be a sign of rising blood urea levels.

Monitoring neurological function requires accurate assessment and correct interpretation of observed data (Bassett & Makin 2000). It is important to take into account the effects of any administered medications, e.g. sedatives and paralysing agents (Woodrow 2000), alcohol consumption, the patient's clinical condition and whether there is a history of head injury.

The aim of this chapter is to understand the principles of monitoring neurological function.

LEARNING OBJECTIVES

At the end of the chapter the reader will be able to:

❑ define *consciousness*;
❑ describe the *AVPU* assessment of consciousness;
❑ discuss the use of the *Glasgow Coma Scale*;
❑ describe *pupillary assessment*;
❑ discuss the principles of *intracranial pressure monitoring*;
❑ discuss the principles of *jugular venous bulb oxygen saturation monitoring*;

❏ outline the monitoring of *sedation*;
❏ outline the monitoring of *pain* and *pain relief*.

DEFINITION OF CONSCIOUSNESS

The patient's level of consciousness has been described as the degree of their arousal and awareness (Chipps *et al.* 1995). It depends on the interaction of the ascending reticular activating system situated in the brainstem and the cerebral hemispheres. Any disruption in this communication process will result in impaired consciousness (Bassett & Makin 2000).

Impaired consciousness in the critically ill patient is usually a neurological expression of a wide range of medical and surgical illnesses (Myburgh & Oh 1997). Definitions of impaired consciousness are listed in Table 4.1. It is not possible

Table 4.1 Definitions of impaired consciousness

Condition	Definition
Consciousness	Awareness of self and environment
Confusion	Reduced awareness, disorientation
Delirium	Disorientation, fear, irritability, misperception, hallucination
Obtundation	Reduced alertness, psychomotor retardation, drowsiness
Stupor	Unresponsiveness with arousal only by vigorous and repeated stimuli
Coma	Unarousable unresponsiveness
Vegetative state	Prolonged coma (>1 month), some preservation of brainstem and motor reflexes
Akinetic mutism	Prolonged coma with apparent alertness and flaccid motor tone
Locked-in state	Total paralysis below third cranial nerve nuclei; normal or impaired mental function

Reproduced with kind permission of Butterworth-Heinemann from Myburgh & Oh 1997 to measure consciousness directly. It can only be assessed by observing the patient's behaviour in response to different stimuli (Shah 1999).

AVPU ASSESSMENT

The most important aspect of any neurological assessment is the level of consciousness because this is the most sensitive guide to cerebral function (Hadfield-Law 1998). A rapid neurological assessment can be carried out using the AVPU method (American College of Surgeons' Committee on Trauma 1997).

AVPU is a mnemonic for a simple, rapid and effective neurological scoring system which quantifies the response to stimulation and assesses the level of consciousness. It is ideal in the emergency situation when a rapid assessment of conscious level is required. AVPU stands for:

*A*lert
responsive to *V*erbal stimulation
responsive to *P*ainful stimulation
*U*nresponsive

THE GLASGOW COMA SCALE

The Glasgow Coma Scale (GCS) was originally developed to grade the severity and outcome of traumatic head injury (Teasdale & Jennett 1974). It is now commonly used to assess the level of consciousness (Mallett & Dougherty 2000) and allows:

- *standardisation* of the clinical observations of patients with impaired consciousness;
- *progress monitoring* of patients undergoing intracranial surgery with minimal variation and subjectivity in the clinical assessment;
- an *indication* to prognosis.

Shah 1999

The Glasgow Coma Scale assesses the two aspects of consciousness:

* *arousal* or *wakefulness*: being aware of the environment;
* *awareness*: demonstrating an understanding of what the practitioner has said through an ability to perform tasks.

The 15-point scale assesses the patient's level of consciousness by evaluating three behavioural responses: eye opening, verbal response and motor response. The best responses are measured (Woodrow 2000). By assigning a numerical value to the level of response to the individual criteria in each section, three figures are obtained which add up to a maximum score of 15. Coma is said to exist when GCS is <8 (Albarran & Price 1998). The lowest possible score is 3 and even a small change in the score may be significant.

Although aggregate scores are often documented, the weighting of scores between eye, verbal and motor responses remains untested (Woodrow 2000). Therefore documenting responses individually may provide a clearer indication of remaining functions and deficits (Watson *et al.* 1992). The neurological observation chart depicted in Fig. 4.1 incorporates the GCS.

The GCS is simple to use, requires no special equipment and is a good predictor of outcome (Woodrow 2000). It can be used by different observers and still produce a consistent assessment, irrespective of a practitioner's status (Juarez & Lyons 1996).

However, as with other scoring systems, the GCS is liable to subjectivity and should only be used as an aid to patient assessment (Adam & Osborne 1999). Intra-observer differences in measuring the GCS may occur (Ellis & Cavenagh 1992). It has therefore been suggested that at shift handover assessment of the patient's GCS by nurses on both shifts should be undertaken in order to identify any discrepancies (Woodrow 2000).

The frequency of GCS monitoring should be individualised

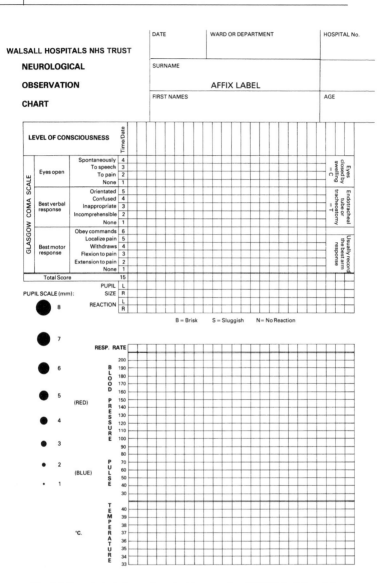

Fig. 4.1 Neurological observation chart incorporating GCS (Walsall Hospitals NHS Trust)

to the patient's needs (Woodrow 2000). Instead of stressing the numerical score attached to each response, it is far better to define the responses in descriptive terms (Myburgh & Oh 1997).

There are difficulties with using the GCS on an ICU (Price 1996), particularly in sedated, ventilated head-injured patients who may also have limb and facial injuries (Ingersoll & Leyden 1987). It only provides an intermittent assessment of consciousness – when a change in one of the parameters causes a deterioration clinically, irreversible damage may already have occurred (McCormick *et al.* 1991).

In addition middle range scores are unreliable (Segatore & Way 1992).

Behavioural responses assessed

The three behavioural responses assessed are:

- eye opening;
- verbal response;
- motor response.

Each will now be discussed in turn.

Eye opening

Assessment of eye opening involves the evaluation of arousal, the first aspect of consciousness. If the patient's eyes are closed, their state of arousal is assessed according to the degree of stimulation required to secure eye opening. Eye opening (arousal) is always the first measurement undertaken as part of the GCS because without it cognition cannot occur (Aucken & Crawford 1998). If the patient's eyes are swollen, opening them may not be possible (Mallett & Dougherty 2000). The scoring is as follows.

- Score 4=spontaneously: eyes open without the need for a stimulus; optimum response.
- Score 3=to speech: eyes open in response to a verbal stimu-

Table 4.2 Central painful stimuli

Trapezium squeeze	Using the thumb and index finger pinch approximately 5 cm of the trapezius muscle (between the head and shoulders) and twist (Woodward 1997)
Suborbital pressure	Running a finger along the supraorbital margin (boney ridge along the top of the eye) it is possible to identify a notch or groove – applying pressure here causes a headache-type pain. Sometimes it may cause the patient to grimace, leading to closing rather than opening of the eyes
	NB should not be used if the patient has facial fractures
Sternal rub	Grinding the sternum with the knuckles

lus (usually the patient's name) which may be normal, loud or repeated.

- Score 2=to pain: eyes open in response to central pain only, e.g. trapezium squeeze, suborbital pressure and pressure in the jaw margin (Table 4.2). **NB** Painful stimuli should only be employed if the patient fails to respond to firm and clear commands (Mallett & Dougherty 2000).
- Score 1=no response: no eye opening despite verbal and central pain stimulus.

NB: record 'C' if the patient is unable to open the eyes due to swelling, ptosis or a dressing.

Verbal response
Assessment of verbal response involves the evaluation of awareness, the second aspect of consciousness. Comprehension of what the practitioner has said (reception of speech) and ability to express thoughts into words (expression of speech) are being evaluated (Shah 1999). Dysphasia or inability to speak can be caused by any damage to the speech centres in the brain, e.g. following intracranial surgery or head injury.

It is important to ascertain the patient's acuity of hearing and understanding of language prior to assessing this response (Adam & Osborne 1999). The lack of speech may not always indicate a falling level of consciousness (Mallett & Dougherty 2000). In addition some patients may require a lot of stimulation to maintain their concentration while answering questions. The amount of stimulation required should be documented as part of baseline assessment (Aucken & Crawford 1998). The scoring is as follows:

- Score 5=orientated: the patient can tell the practitioner who they are, where they are and the day, date and year (Aucken & Crawford 1998).
- Score 4=confused: the patient can hold a conversation with the practitioner, but can not answer questions accurately.
- Score 3=inappropriate words: the patient may say some words but they are said at random or are inappropriate.
- Score 2=incomprehensible sounds: the patient's response is made up of incomprehensible sounds, but no discernible words. A verbal stimulus together with a pain stimulus may be needed to get a response from the patient.
- Score 1=no response: no response from the patient despite both verbal and pain stimuli.

NB: record 'D' if the patient is dysphasic and 'T' if the patient has a tracheal or tracheostomy tube.

Motor response

The motor response is designed to ascertain the patient's ability to obey a command and to localise, withdraw or assume abnormal body positions in response to a painful stimulus (Adam & Osborne 1999). If the patient does not respond by obeying commands the response to a painful stimulus should then be assessed.

In the past the application of a peripheral painful stimulus (pressure applied to fingernail bed) has been advocated (Teasdale & Jennett 1974). However this can be traumatic and is no longer recommended. In addition a peripheral stimulus may only elicit a spinal reflex which does not involve cerebral function (Shah 1999). It can cause patients to pull their fingers away from the source of pain; only a central painful stimulus will demonstrate localisation to pain (Hickey 1997).

A true localising response involves the patient bringing an arm up to chin level. To elicit this response the trapezium squeeze, supraorbital pressure or pressure on the jaw margin are recommended. To avoid soft tissue injury no stimulus should be applied for more than 30 s (Bassett & Makin 2000). In addition, when applying a stimulus, it is best practice to start off with light pressure and increase to elicit a response (Sheppard & Wright 2000).

- Score 6=obeys commands: ask the patient to stick his tongue out; never ask a patient just to squeeze your hand as this could elicit a primitive grasp response which could be confused with an appropriate response (Woodward 1997). As it is important to establish that the response is not just a reflex movement, it is important to ask the patient to carry out two different commands (Bassett & Makin 2000).
- Score 5=localises to pain: the patient purposely moves an arm in an attempt to remove the cause of the pain. The patient may also localise in attempting to remove something that is uncomfortable or irritable, e.g. nasogastric tube (Woodward 1997).
- Score 4=withdrawing from pain: the patient flexes or bends arm towards the source of the pain but makes no attempt to remove the source of the pain. There is no wrist rotation. Hemiparesis or hemiplegia may be evident if both arms do not flex equally (Woodward 1997).
- Score 3=flexion to pain: the patient flexes or bends the arm at the elbow and rotates the wrist resulting in a 'spastic' posture (Shah 1999). It indicates abnormal nerve pathway function (Hickey 1997) and is sometimes referred to as decorticate movement.

- Score 2=extension to pain: the patient extends the arm by straightening the elbow, sometimes associated with internal shoulder and hand rotation (Woodward 1997). Sometimes referred to as decerebrate movement.
- Score 1=no response: no response to central painful stimuli.

Application of painful stimuli

Best practice – application of painful stimuli

Painful stimuli should only be employed if the patient fails to respond to firm and clear commands

To evaluate cerebral function, apply a central not peripheral stimulus, e.g. trapezium squeeze, supraorbital pressure or pressure on the jaw margin

When applying a stimulus, start off with light pressure and increase to elicit a response

To avoid soft tissue injury no stimulus should be applied for more than 30 s

---

PUPILLARY ASSESSMENT

Although pupillary assessment is not part of the GCS, it is an essential adjunct to it. Any changes in pupil reaction, size or shape, together with other neurological signs, are a late sign of raised intracranial pressure (Woodward 1997).

Prior to undertaking pupillary assessment the following should be noted:

- any pre-existing irregularity with the pupils, e.g. cataracts, false eye and previous eye injury;
- factors that cause pupillary dilation, e.g. medications including tricyclics, atropine and sympathomimetics and traumatic mydriasis (Myburgh & Oh 1997);
- factors that cause pupillary constriction, e.g. medications including narcotics and topical beta-blockers.
  Pupillary assessment should include the following observations.

- *Size* (mm): prior to shining light into the eyes, estimate pupil size using the scale printed on the neurological assessment chart as a comparison. The average size is 2–5mm (Shah 1999). Both pupils should be equal in size.
- *Shape*: should be round; abnormal shapes may indicate cerebral damage; oval shape indicates coning (Hickey 1997).
- *Reactivity to light*: a bright light source (usully a pen torch) should be moved from the outer aspect of the eye towards the pupil – a brisk pupil constriction should ensue (Smith 1998). Following removal of the light source the pupil should return to its original size. The procedure should be repeated for the other eye. There should also be a consensual reaction to the light source, i.e. both eyes constrict when the light source is applied to the one. Unreactive pupils can be caused by an expanding mass, e.g. a blood clot exerting pressure on the 3rd cranial nerve; a fixed and dilated pupil may be due to herniation of the medial temporal lobe (Bassett & Makin 2000). The reaction should be documented (Fig. 4.1) as '+' or B for brisk, – or 'N' for no reaction and sl or S for some or sluggish reaction (follow local policy). **NB** lens implants or cataracts may prevent the pupil from constricting to light (Aucken & Crawford 1998).
- *Equality*: both pupils should be the same shape, size and react equally to light.

PRINCIPLES OF INTRACRANIAL PRESSURE MONITORING

Intracranial pressure (ICP) is the pressure exerted by the normal cerebral components (brain, blood and cerebral spinal fluid) within the rigid structure of the skull. ICP monitoring measures the pressure within the skull exerted by these components (Rutherford & Nelson 1995).

A raised ICP occurs when one of the skull components increases in volume, thus displacing brain tissue, blood or cerebral spinal fluid (Bassett & Makin 2000). This can lead to a fall in cerebral perfusion pressure resulting in reduced cerebral perfusion and inadequate oxygen delivery.

Early detection of a raised ICP is therefore essential in order to prevent increasing cerebral damage and death. By inserting an ICP bolt or an intraventricular catheter, ICP can be continually monitored. The normal ICP is 10–15 mmHg; an ICP of > 20 mmHg is a cause for concern (Rutherford & Nelson 1995).

Vital signs

It is important to monitor the patient's vital signs because they can be dramatically affected by a rise in intracranial pressure. The centres controlling heart rate, blood pressure, respiration and temperature are located in the brainstem.

Of these four vital signs, the monitoring of respirations provides the clearest indication of cerebral function because they are controlled by different areas of the brain (Mallett & Dougherty 2000). The rate, character and pattern of respirations must be noted. Abnormal patterns in respirations have been discussed in Chapter 1.

A rising blood pressure and falling heart rate and respiratory rate are signs of increased intracranial pressure (Cushing's reflex) (Nikas 1982). A sudden massive rise in intracranial pressure, e.g. following a large subarachnoid haemorrhage, can cause a Cheyne Stokes breathing pattern (Shah 1999). Damage to the hypothalamus can cause changes in temperature.

Indications

Indications for ICP monitoring include:

- requirement for mechanical ventilation;
- GCS score of <8: approximately two thirds of patients with head injuries with a GCS of 8 or less develop elevated ICP (Becker 1989);
- presence of small haematoma seen on the CT scan;
- after decompression surgery.

Hinds & Watson 1996

ICP bolt

The bolt is inserted by a small twist. Bolts generally measure subdural pressure (Sutcliffe 1997) and monitor traces may be dampened and unreliable (Waldmann & Thyveetil 1998). Complications are rare. The risk of meningitis is reduced because the ventricle is not penetrated (Hickman *et al.* 1990).

Intraventricular catheter

This is the gold standard for ICP monitoring (Menon 1997). Connection to a transducer permits visible tracings on a monitor. In addition the catheter may be connected to a drainage system, allowing drainage by gravity if the ICP exceeds a set level, thus allowing nurses to maintain the pressure within normal parameters.

Once the catheter is positioned it should be marked with permanent ink to facilitate the recognition of tube migration. Complications include infection and haemorrhage (Eddy *et al.* 1995).

Maintaining accuracy

It is important to:

• maintain the transducer at the same level as the foramen of Monro or at the level of the ear;
• zero balance and recalibrate whenever the patient's position is altered;
• ensure air bubbles do not enter the transducer or tubing as this could dampen the trace and cause inaccurate ICP measurements.

Valenti *et al.* 1997

Inaccurate or misleading measurements are the most common pitfalls encountered with ICP monitoring (Bergsneider & Becker 1995).

PRINCIPLES OF JUGULAR VENOUS BULB OXYGEN SATURATION MONITORING

This advanced form of monitoring is being increasingly used in neuroscience units, particularly for patients with head injuries. In combination with other clinical signs and physiological variables it enables the detection of cerebral ischaemia, provides a useful guide to more differentiated therapy and is prognostically accurate (Moore & Knowles 1999).

A fibre-optic catheter is inserted into the internal jugular vein and threaded upwards to the jugular bulb. Contra-indications to insertion include significant trauma to the neck, a hypercoagulable state and bleeding diathesis (Moore & Knowles 1999).

Jugular venous bulb oxygen saturation monitoring (SjO_2) provides an indication to global cerebral oxygen delivery, but not regional ischaemia (Feldman & Robertson 1997). Cerebral oxygen consumption is usually 35–40% of available oxygen; the normal SjO_2 is therefore 60–65% (March 1994).

Changes in SjO_2 are reflective of changes in cerebral metabolic rate and cerebral blood flow (Woodrow 2000). A reading below 50% for > 15 min has been described as a jugular desaturation episode (Dearden 1991) and is associated with a poor neurological outcome (Gopinath *et al*. 1994). It should be noted that falls in SjO_2 can lag behind a rise in ICP and the clinical signs of deterioration (Sheinberg *et al*. 1992).

SjO_2 monitoring shares many of the problems encountered with pulse oximetry (Woodrow 2000). Almost half of the apparent desaturation episodes are caused by technical problems, e.g. low light intensity (Sikes & Segal 1994). Light density should be monitored to ensure the accuracy of the readings.

Causes of high and low SjO_2

Causes of high SjO_2 (>80%) include:

- a rise in cerebral blood flow;
- a fall in oxygen extraction;

- raised ICP;
- hyperventilation.

Sikes & Segal 1994

Causes of low SjO_2 (<50%) include:

- hypoxia;
- hypotension and cerebral hypoperfusion.

High SjO_2 may reflect a fall in cerebral metabolic demand for oxygen, e.g. tissue death, hyopthermia or the use of medications such as thiopentone; in fact an initial low SjO_2 followed by a gradual rise to >75% may be a preterminal event indicating initial ischaemia and then death of cerebral tissue (Moore & Knowles 1999).

PRINCIPLES OF MONITORING SEDATION

The purpose of sedation is to allow the patient to sleep undisturbed, minimise discomfort, abolish pain, reduce anxiety and facilitate organ-system support and nursing care (Bion & Oh 1997). Where possible the patient should still be able to communicate coherently, though in some situations, e.g. raised intracranial pressure deeper sedation will be required.

Effects of over- and under-sedation

Over-sedation deprives the patient of life awareness and can cause respiratory and cardiovascular depression. Under-sedation exposes the patient to noxious stimuli, e.g. pain; increased protein breakdown from stress-induced hypermetabolism prolongs the process of weaning from the ventilator (Woodrow 2000) resulting in prolonged bed rest increasing the risk of immobility complications. Sedation should therefore be accurately assessed.

Assessment of sedation

It is difficult to assess sedation because the needs of patients vary (Shelly 1998) and discrepancies between practitioners' assessment exists (Westcott 1995). Haemodynamic changes are unreliable because most ICU patients are already labile (Shelly 1998).

As corneal reflexes remain until the patient is in a deep coma (Myburgh & Oh 1997), gently brushing the tips of the patient's eyelashes as a method of assessing whether the patient is sufficiently sedated to tolerate traumatic interventions, such as intubation, has been suggested (Woodrow 2000).

Bion and Oh (1997) suggest the following methods of assessing sedation.

- *Level of consciousness* (or depth of sedation): to include any pain or discomfort, comprehension, tolerance of organ-system support and illness severity. There are various sedation scales currently in use, e.g. the Ramsey sedation scale (Ramsey *et al.* 1974) (Table 4.3).
- Linear analogue scales: when recorded by trained observers, these allow the various components of sedation to be measured independently. They are descriptively flexible and can be analysed either graphically or numerically (Wallace *et al.* 1988).

Problems associated with sedation

Problems associated with sedation include:

- hypotension;
- prevention of sleep;
- amnesia (Perrins *et al.* 1998).

Table 4.3 The Ramsey sedation scale

Awake levels

(1) Patient anxious and agitated or restless or both
(2) Patient cooperative, orientated and tranquil
(3) Patient responds to command only

Asleep levels

(4) Brisk response
(5) Sluggish response
(6) No response

Source: Ramsey *et al.* 1974

It is also important to be familiar with the specific side-effects of the analgesics or hypnotics used for sedation.

Monitoring pain and pain relief

For the purpose of this book only some basic principles of monitoring pain and pain relief will be discussed. If the reader requires more in-depth information, there are books available that are dedicated to the subject of pain management, e.g. McCaffery and Beebe (1994).

Causes of pain

The patient may have acute pain, e.g. following surgery or chronic pain, e.g. osteoarthritis. A post discharge survey of ICU patients carried out by Puntillo (1990) found that the following caused moderate to severe pain:

- surgery;
- intubation;
- removal of chest drains;
- suction;
- potassium infusions.

In the critical care environment pain is aggravated by anxiety, fear, communication difficulties and the need for life-saving interventions (Adam & Osborne 1999).

Assessing pain

Sometimes assessing pain in critically ill patients can be difficult, particularly if they are intubated, sedated or have impaired psychomotor skills (Woodrow 2000). Pain is often inadequately assessed in critically ill patients (Puntillo 1990). In these situations physiological variables, e.g. tachycardia, a rise in blood pressure and physical responses, e.g. sweating and facial expression are particularly important (Adam & Osborne 1999).

The use of pain assessment tools improves pain control

(Scott 1994), though unfortunately there is currently no ideal ICU pain assessment tool (Woodrow 2000).

Relieving/preventing pain

The pioneering research carried out by Hayward (1975) demonstrated that preparation and honest explanations reduce pain, analgesia requirements and recovery time. Good communication is essential.

Methods of pain relief include analgesia, e.g. opiates, regional analgesia, e.g. epidurals and nitrous oxide. Following administration of the chosen pain relief, it is important to evaluate its effectiveness. Although this should be common sense, nurses often fail to do this (Tittle & McMillan 1994).

The use of a pain chart or of adequate recording in the patient's care plan is important if pain relief intervention is to be properly evaluated (Adam & Osborne 1999). It is also important to be alert to the possible side effects of pain relief, e.g. respiratory depression following opiate administration.

Epidural analgesia

Epidural analgesia is widely used postoperatively (Audit Commission 1997). A catheter is placed in the epidural space and analgesia, e.g. diamorphine, fentanyl and an anesthetic, e.g. 0.125% bupivacaine can be administered either continuously through an infusion or by bolus injections. The insertion site should be checked for leaks, signs of skin irritation and infection (Chapman & Day 2001). Close monitoring of the patient is essential to identify any complications which could include:

- respiratory depression;
- hypotension;
- nausea and vomiting;
- urinary retention due to inhibition of the micturition reflex;
- catheter migration.

Chapman & Day 2001

The following parameters should be monitored:

- vital signs;
- sedation score;
- pain score;
- fluid balance;
- level/depth of block.

Hall 2000.

Scenario

A 25-year-old man is admitted to A & E with a head injury after falling off his bicycle. He is fully conscious, talking to you and there are no obvious injuries. What are your initial monitoring priorities?

The airway is clear and the neck is immobilised in case of cervical spinal injury. BP 120/70, resps 15, pulse 90, SpO₂ 98%, GCS 15; pupils are medium and both reacting equally and briskly to light. A CT scan is ordered. What on-going monitoring will the patient require?

The patient's vital signs, SpO₂, GCS and pupillary assessment continue to be monitored. The patient starts to demonstrate signs of confusion. BP 120/75, pulse 94, SpO₂ 97%, GCS 13; pupils are medium and both reacting equally and briskly to light. What can be deducted from these observations?

The patient's vital signs are stable, but the slight drop in the GCS is of concern. The patient is taken for a CT scan. During the procedure his conscious level falls dramatically. BP 170/100, pulse 55, resps 10, SpO₂ 96%, GCS 9. He is responding and localising to pain and making incomprehensible sounds. His right pupil is dilated and not reacting to light. The left pupil is medium and reacting briskly to light. What can be deduced from these observations?

A right sided subdural haematoma is confirmed by the CT scan. A rise in BP, fall in heart and respiratory rates and the deterioration in conscious level are signs consistent with a raised intracranial pressure. The problem with the right pupil is consistent with the right sided subdural lesion. Urgent neurosurgical referral is required. Ongoing monitoring must continue with particular attention to the maintenance of a clear airway.

CONCLUSION

Monitoring neurological function is central to the care of all critically ill patients, particularly those with a head injury or other cerebral insult. It enables the early recognition and treatment of complications and can improve prognosis. It can also provide an indication to the function of other major systems in the body. The administration of medications, e.g. sedatives and paralysing agents and any recent alcohol consumption should be taken into account.

REFERENCES

Adam, S. & Osborne, S. (1999) *Critical Care Nursing: Science and Practice*. Oxford Medical Publications, Oxford.

Albarran, J. & Price, T. (1998) *Managing the Nursing Priorities in Intensive Care*. Quay Books/Mark Allen Publishing, Dinton.

American College of Surgeons' Committee on Trauma (1997) *Student Course Manual*. American College of Surgeons, Chicago.

Aucken, S. & Crawford, B. (1998) Neurological assessment. In: D. Guerrero, ed. *Neuro-Oncology for Nurses*. Whurr Publishers, London.

Audit Commission (1997) *Anaesthesia Under Examination*. The Stationery Office, London.

Bassett, C. & Makin, L., eds (2000) *Caring for the Seriously Ill Patient*. Arnold, London.

Becker, D. (1989) Common themes in head injury. In: D. Becker & S. Gudeman, eds. *Textbook of. Head Injury*. W.B. Saunders, Philadelphia.

Bergsneider, M. & Becker, D. (1995) Intracranial pressure monitoring. In: S. Ayres, A. Grenvik, P. Holbrook & W. Shoemaker eds, *Textbook of Critical Care* 3rd edn. W.B. Saunders, London.

Bion, J. & Oh, T. (1997) Sedation in intensive care. In: T. Oh, ed. *Intensive Care Manual*, 4th edn. Butterworth Heinemann, Oxford.

Chapman, S. & Day, R. (2001) Spinal anatomy and the use of epidurals. *Professional Nurse* **16** (6), 1174–1177.

Chipps, E. M. *et al.* (1995) *Neurologic Disorders* Mosby's Clinical Nursing Series Vol 6. C.V. Mosby Co, St Louis.

Closs, S. (1992) Patients' night-time pain, analgesia provision and sleep after surgery. *International Journal of Nursing Studies* **29** (4), 381–392.

Dearden, N. (1991) Jugular venous oxygen saturation in the management of severe head injury. *Current Opinions in Anaesthesiology* **4**, 279–296.

Eddy, V., Vitsky, J., Rutherford, E. *et al.* (1995) Aggressive use of ICP monitoring is safe and alters patient care. *American Surgery* **61** (1), 24–29.

Ellis, A. & Cavenagh, S. (1992) Aspects of neurosurgical assessment using the Glasgow Coma Scale. *Intensive and Critical Care Nursing* **8** (2), 94–99.

Feldman, Z. & Robertson, C. (1997) Monitoring of cerebral haemodynamics with jugular bulb catheters. *Critical Care Clinics* **13**(1), 51–77.

Gopinath, S., Robertson, C., Contant, C. *et al.* (1994) Jugular venous desaturation and outcome after head injury. *Journal of Neurological and Neurosurgical Psychiatry* **57**, 717–723.

Hadfield-Law, L. (1998) Life and death decisions. *Nursing Times* **94** (41), 24–26.

Hall, J. (2000) Epidural analgesia management. *Nursing Times* **96** (28), 38–40.

Hayward, J. (1975) *Information: A Prescription Against Pain*. RCN, London.

Hickey, J. (1997) Intracranial pressure: theory and management of intracranial pressure. In: J. Hickey, ed. *The Clinical Practice of Neurological and Neurosurgical Nursing* 4th edn. Lippincott, Philadelphia.

Hickman, K., Mayer, B. & Muswases, M. (1990) Intracranical pressure monitoring: review of risk factors associated with infection. *Heart and Lung* **19** (1), 84–89.

Hinds, C.J. & Watson, D. (1996) *Intensive Care. A Concise Textbook*, 2nd edn. W.B. Saunders, London.

Ingersoll, G. & Leyden, D. (1987) The Glasgow Coma Scale for patients with head injuries. *Critical Care Nurse* **7** (5), 26–32.

Juarez, V. & Lyons, M. (1996) Inter-rater reliability of the Glasgow Coma Scale. *Journal of Neuroscience Nursing* **27** (5), 283–286.

McCaffery, M. & Beebe, A. (1994) *Pain: Clinical Manual for Nursing Practice*. C.V. Mosby, London.

McCormick, P., Stewart, M., Goetting, M. *et al.* (1991) Non-invasive cerebral optical spectroscopy for monitoring cerebral oxygen delivery and haemodynamics. *Critical Care Medicine* **19** (1), 89-97.

Mallett, J. & Dougherty, L. (2000), eds. *The Royal Marsden Hospital Manual of Clinical Nursing Procedures*. Blackwell Science, Oxford.

March, K. (1994) Retrograde jugular catheter: monitoring SjO$_2$. *Journal of Neuroscience Nursing* **26** (1), 48–51.

Menon, D. (1997) Monitoring the central nervous system. *Current Anaesthesia and Critical Care* **8** (6), 254–263.

Moore, P. & Knowles, M. (1999) Jugular venous bulb oxygen saturation monitoring in neuro critical care. *Care of the Critically Ill* **15** (5), 163–166.

Myburgh, J. & Oh, T. (1997) Disorders of consciousness. In: T. Oh, ed. *Intensive Care Manual*, 4th edn. Butterworth Heinemann, Oxford.

Nelson, L.D. & Rutherford, E.J. (1993) Principles of hemodynamic monitoring. In: M.R. Pinsky & J.F. Dhainaut, eds. *Pathophysiologic Foundations of Critical Care*. Williams & Wilkins, Baltimore.

Nikas, D., ed. (1982) *The Critically Ill Neurosurgical Patient*. Churchill Livingstone, New York.

Perrins, J., King, N. & Collings, J. (1998) Assessment of long-term psychological well-being following intensive care. *Intensive and Critical Care Nursing* **14** (3), 108–116.

Phillips, G. (1997) Pain relief in intensive care. In: T. Oh, ed. *Intensive Care Manual*, 4th edn. Butterworth Heinemann, Oxford.

Price, T. (1996) An evaluation of neuro-assessment tools in the intensive care unit. *Nursing and Critical Care* **1** (2), 72–77.

Puntillo, K. (1990) The phenomenon of pain and critical care nursing. *Heart and Lung* **17** (5), 526–533.

Ramsey, M., Savage, T., Simpson, B. *et al.* (1974) Controlled sedation with alphaxalone and alphadolone. *British Medical Journal* **2**, 656–659.

Rutherford, E. & Nelson, L. (1995) Initial assessment of multiple trauma patients. In: S. Ayres, A. Grenvik, P. Holbrook & W. Shoemaker eds, *Textbook of Critical Care* 3rd edn. W.B. Saunders, London.

Scott, I. (1994) Effectiveness of documented assessment. *Nursing Standard* **3** (10), 494–501.

Segatore, M. & Way, C. (1992) The Glasgow Coma Scale: time for change. *Heart and Lung* **21** (6), 548–557.

Shah, S. (1999) Neurological assessment. *Nursing Standard* **13** (22), 49–54.

Sheinberg, M., Kanter, M., Robertson, C. *et al.* (1992) Continuous monitoring of jugular venous oxygen saturation in head injured patients. *Journal of Neurosurgery* **76**, 212–217.

Shelly, M. (1994) Assessing sedation. *Care of the Critically Ill* **10** (3), 118–121.

Shelly, M. (1998) Sedation in the ITU. *Care of the Critically Ill* **14** (3), 85–88.

Sheppard, M. & Wright, M. (2000) *High Dependency Nursing*. Ballière-Tindall, London.

Sikes, P. & Segal, J. (1994) Jugular venous bulb oxygen saturation monitoring for evaluating cerebral ischaemia. *Critical Care Nursing Quarterly* **17** (1), 9–20.

Silk, D. (1994) *Organisation of Nutritional Support in Hospitals*. BAPEN, London.

Smith, I. (1998) Eye care 1: external examination: practical procedures for nurses. *Nursing Times* **94** (37), Suppl. 1–2.

Sutcliffe, J. (1997) Assessment of cerebral function. In: D. Goldhill & P. Withington eds, *Textbook of Intensive Care*. Chapman & Hall, London.

Teasdale, G. & Jennett, B. (1974) Assessment of coma and impaired consciousness: a practical scale. *The Lancet* **2**, 81–84.

Tittle, M. & McMillan, S. (1994) Pain and pain-related side effects in an ICU and on a surgical unit: nurse's management. *American Journal of Critical Care* **3**, 25–30.

Valenti, L., Tamblyn, R. & Rozinski, M.B. (1997) *Critical Care Nursing*. J B Lippincott, New York.

Waldmann, C. & Thyveetil, D. (1998) Management of head injury in a district general hospital. *Care of the Critically Ill* **14** (2), 65–70.

Wallace, P., Bion, J. & Ledingham, I. (1998) The changing face of sedative practice. In: I. Ledingham, ed., *Recent Advances in Critical Care Medicine*. Churchill Livingstone, Edinburgh.

Watson, M. *et al.* (1992) Searching for signs of revival. *Professional Nurse* **7** (10), 670–674.

Westcott, C. (1995) The sedation of patients in intensive care units. *Intensive and Critical Care Nursing* **11** (1), 26-31.

Woodrow, P. (2000) *Intensive Care Nursing: A Framework for Practice*. Routledge, London.

Woodward, S. (1997) Neurological observations – 1 Glasgow Coma Scale. *Nursing Times* **93** (45), Suppl. 1–2.

Monitoring Renal Function

5

INTRODUCTION

The renal function should be closely monitored in all critically ill patients. First, it can provide an indication of the function of other systems, e.g. the cardiovascular system, where a low cardiac output will result in a diminished urine output. Second, the early recognition and prompt treatment of acute renal failure is essential if prognosis is to be maximised. Patients receiving renal replacement therapy should also be closely monitored.

The aim of this chapter is to understand the principles of monitoring renal function.

LEARNING OBJECTIVES

At the end of the chapter the reader will be able to:

❏ describe the principles of *urinalysis*;
❏ discuss the principles of *urine output monitoring*;
❏ outline the key principles of monitoring *fluid balance*;
❏ discuss the management of *acute renal failure*;
❏ outline aspects of *management*;
❏ outline the key aspects of *monitoring during renal replacement therapy*.

PRINCIPLES OF URINALYSIS

> 'This valuable fluid should not be discarded in any patient in whom a renal, diabetic, gastrointestinal or other major system disease is suspected.'
>
> (Talley & O'Connor 1998)

Urinalysis can provide important information that can assist in diagnosis and can help in the monitoring of a patient's clinical condition. It must be emphasised however, that the findings can not be interpreted in isolation in order to provide a nursing and medical diagnosis: they should only be used as part of a full and detailed assessment including physical, psychological and social factors (Torrance 1998). The appearance and odour of the urine should also be noted.

Appearance of urine

Normal urine is straw coloured and clear, but becomes turbid when left to stand. Variations in the appearance of urine include the following.

- *Pale*: urine is dilute; causes include overhydration, diabetes mellitus or insipidus and polyuria in renal disease resulting from the tubules failing to reabsorb water.
- *Dark*: urine is concentrated as seen in fluid depletion or contains bile.
- *Orange*: usually caused by specific drugs, e.g. rifampicin.
- *Pink/red*: may indicate haematuria, though other causes include ingestion of certain foodstuffs, e.g. beetroot.
- *Cloudy*: may indicate infection.
- *Debris*: may indicate infection.
- *Frothy*: may indicate significant proteinuria.

Odour

Normal, freshly voided urine is practically odourless. If left to stand for several hours it acquires a mild smell of ammonia. Infected urine has a 'fishy' smell. In diabetic patients with ketoacidosis or in patients who are anorexic or are not eating, acetone is excreted in the urine causing the urine to smell characteristically sweet.

Urinary incontinence

Urinary incontinence can occur transiently. Causes include urinary tract infections, delirium, excess urine output, e.g. following diuretics, faeces impaction and immobility (patient unable to reach the toilet or use a urinal) and spinal cord compression (necessitating emergency surgery).

Procedure for dipstick test of urine

A dipstick test of urine can accurately show the presence of a variety of substances, e.g. protein, glucose, ketones and blood, as well as the pH. To ensure reliable results, the following procedure for dipstick urine testing is recommended.

- Check the expiry date on the container, ensuring the testing strips are in date.
- Remove a testing strip from the container and replace the cap straight away.
- Dip the testing strip into a fresh sample of urine, ensuring all the reagent pads of the strip are covered. The urine must be fresh because 'stored' urine rapidly deteriorates which can cause false results (Mallett & Dougherty 2000).
- Wipe off any excess urine on the rim of the specimen container.
- Place the testing strip flat on a dry surface to prevent the urine from running from square to square resulting in reagents mixing together. This may lead to an inaccurate result.
- Compare the reagent pads with the colour scale at time intervals stipulated by the manufacturer. If the strips are not read at the exactly the time intervals specified, the reagents may not have had time to react which could cause inaccurate results (Mallett & Dougherty 2000).
- Discard the urine sample and used testing strip.
- Record the results in the patient's notes and report any abnormalities.

It is essential to store and use the reagent strips correctly, following the manufacturer's recommendations, in order to ensure accurate and reliable results. The package insert supplied by the manufacturers will contain detailed instructions which normally include the following general points:

- the reagent strip should be stored in the container supplied by the manufacturer;
- the container cap should be replaced as soon as the reagent strip has been removed;
- the desiccant should never be removed from the bottle – some manufacturers incorporate it into the lid of the container so that it can not be lost;
- the container should be stored in a cool dry place, but not refrigerated;
- reagent strips should not be used after the expiry date on the container (note that the expiry date may refer to the shelf life of an unopened container or an opened 'in use' container (Cook 1996)).

Some drugs can influence urinalysis, e.g. high does of aspirin can cause a false negative reaction to glycosuria (Mallett & Dougherty 2000). It is therefore paramount to take into account the patient's medication when examining the results of dipstick urinalysis.

Best practice – urinalysis

Always use a fresh sample of urine

Observe sample for colour, appearance, smell and debris

Ensure reagent strip is in date

Ensure whole of reagent strip is immersed in urine sample

Wipe off excess urine, place horizontal and compare reagent pads with colour scale at time intervals stipulated by manufacturer and document results immediately

Safely discard strip and urine sample

Store reagent strips following manufacturer's recommendations

---

Significance of the results

Glycosuria is due to abnormally high blood glucose levels and can be associated with stress, diabetes mellitus, acute pancreatitis, Cushing's syndrome and steroid therapy.

Ketones (ketonuria) are suggestive of excessive fat breakdown as in starvation or excessive dieting and uncontrolled diabetes mellitus.

Proteinuria is the presence of abnormally large quantities of protein, usually albumin (it is sometimes therefore termed albuminuria). Normally, no more than a trace of protein should be found in urine (250 mg protein in 24 h), though sometimes a dipstick test may only show positive if the protein levels are 1.5 g or above in 24 h (Smith 1998).

Persistent proteinuria is usually a sign of renal disease, e.g. urinary tract infection, pyelonephritis or a renal complication of another disease, e.g. hypertension, congestive cardiac failure and pre-eclampsia. Sometimes proteinuria can be associated with strenuous exercise or pyrexia.

The presence of blood (haematuria) may be caused by trauma, catheter trauma, infection, renal stones and drugs.

Bilirubin (bilirubinuria) may indicate hepatic or biliary disease. False positive results may be obtained if stale urine specimens are used (Torrance & Elley 1997).

Raised levels of urobilonogen may indicate hepatic disease or excessive haemolysis, e.g. in haemolytic anaemia.

The presence of haemoglobin (haemoglobinuria) is suggestive of a reaction to a blood transfusion, haemolytic anaemia or severe burns (Mallett & Dougherty 2000).

Nitrites in urine may indicate a urinary tract infection.

Leucocytes (pyuria) in urine are suggestive of a urinary tract infection, but follow-up urine culture is required.

The pH of normal urine is 6 (slightly acidotic), but the pH can range from 4.0 to 8.0 in cases of severe acidosis or alkalosis, respectively (Smith 1998).

The specific gravity of urine is a measure of the ability of the kidneys to dilute or concentrate urine (Cook 1996). A high specific gravity may indicate dehydration while a low one may indicate overhydration, renal abnormalities or diabetes inspidus.

Other urine tests

Osmolality
Measurement of osmolality indicates the ability of the kidneys to concentrate and dilute the urine. It is considered more accurate than measuring specific gravity (Smith 1998).

Creatinine clearance
The principle of clearance is that an estimation of a known substance (which is only excreted in the urine) in the plasma is compared with the amount in the urine. Creatinine is produced by the breakdown of creatinine phosphate, which is manufactured by the muscle mass at a fairly constant rate. It is present in the circulation and is filtered by the glomeruli. The normal value for creatinine clearance is 70–125 ml/min and a result of <10 ml/min is an indication for starting renal replacement therapy (Smith 1998).

As creatinine clearance is at its highest in the afternoon (Sladen 1994), a 24 h urine collection is therefore necessary to ensure accuracy of measurement. At the same time a blood sample is taken to establish the concurrent levels of creatinine in the plasma.

Microscopy and culture
Being the most concentrated, the first voided urine of the day is the best for culture. Ideally the sample should be taken before starting a broad spectrum antibiotic, which may be given in the interim period before a specific sensitivity is identified.

URINE OUTPUT MONITORING
Although urine output is only an index to renal perfusion, it is frequently used as a guide to the adequacy of cardiac output (renal perfusion amounts to 25% of the cardiac output).

However the use of diuretics, such as frusemide or dopamine, abolishes its value as a haemodynamic monitor (Gomersall & Oh 1997).

Urine is composed of 95% water and 5% solids, mainly urea and sodium chloride; it is slightly acidic (pH 6.0) and has a specific gravity of 1.010–1.030 (SG of water is 1.000) (Smith 1998). The average urine output in a healthy adult is 1000–1500 ml per day. Listed below are the generally accepted rates of urine production associated with urinary output disorders:

- anuria: <50 ml of urine in 24 h;
- oliguria: <400 ml of urine in 24 h;
- polyuria: >3000 ml of urine in 24 h;
- painful micturition is known as dysuria.

Talley and O'Connor (1998)

All critically ill patients will require a urinary catheter. If urine output measurements are required the patient should be catheterised and an hourly urine drainage bag attached (Fig. 5.1). The urinary catheter should be closely monitored because it can become blocked, e.g. from a blood clot or become occluded, e.g. due to kinking. Sometimes bladder washouts are indicated if difficulties with drainage are encountered.

MONITORING FLUID BALANCE

Monitoring fluid balance in the critically ill patient is paramount. Physiological mechanisms, disease processes and treatment side-effects are just a few of the numerous factors that can affect fluid status (Sheppard 2000). Fluid and electrolyte overload is sometimes difficult to avoid and is commonly found in patients with multiple organ failure (Gosling 1999).

Careful monitoring of the fluid balance chart must be maintained and this should include all input and output. Monitoring the patient for signs of fluid loss/gain should also be undertaken and Table 5.1 provides an overview of this. The

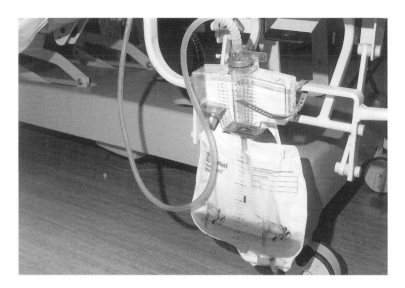

Fig. 5.1 Hourly urine drainage bag

importance of monitoring urine output, urine osmolality and specific gravity of urine have already been discussed.

Daily measurement of serum sodium, potassium, urea and creatinine together with 24h urine volume are required to assess fluid and electrolyte balance. In addition, fluid balance charts from the preceding few days should be compared to serum and urine urea and electrolyte values. This will help evaluate the patient's response to fluid administration and will guide the fluid regime over the next 12–24h (Gosling 1999). The nature and volume of any fluid replacement therapy will depend on fluid loss (Sheppard 2000).

MANAGEMENT OF ACUTE RENAL FAILURE

Acute renal failure (ARF) can be defined as a sudden deterioration in renal function that results in the inability to excrete

Table 5.1 Systemic signs and symptoms of fluid loss and gain

System	Signs in fluid loss	Signs in fluid gain	Monitoring and nursing observation
Cardiovascular	Increase heart rate Irregular thready pulse Reduced blood pressure and CVP	Increased heart rate, BP, CVP Neck vein distension may be evident	Pulse Blood pressure CVP
Respiratory	Increased respiratory rate Hyperventilation	Increased rate Dyspnoea and pulmonary oedema may be evident	Nature and frequency of respirations Signs of waterlogging of pulmonary circulation Oxygenation status–skin colour Saturation, i.e. pulse oximetry/ blood gases
Urinary system	Urine output decreased, or increased in diabetes insipidus	Output may be increased or decreased depending on the underlying cause and renal function	Volume of urine output/24 h period.
General orientation	Apprehension Restlessness	Confusion Irritability	General orientation status
Skin	Texture is dry and lax, under-perfusion of tissues and reduced vascularity leading to skin colour change, dry mucous membranes and evidence of thirst Excessive perspiration accompanies increased body temperature	Dependent, generalised, and/or pitting oedema The skin may be warm, moist and swollen with the appearance of being tight and shiny	General appearance/ hydrational status Colour Temperature Condition of mucous membranes

Reprinted by permission of Baillière Tindall from Sheppard & Wright (2000)

the products of metabolism resulting in a rise in blood urea and other nitrogen waste products (Toto 1992).

Inadequate renal perfusion resulting from a serious insult, e.g. haemorrhage, burns, sepsis and trauma which has resulted in circulatory shock, is the commonest cause of ARF on the intensive care unit (Bellomo 1997 and Hamilton 1999). ARF can also result from a single identifiable event such as drug toxicity (Hinds & Watson 1996).

ARF can be classified into three groups.

- *Prerenal*: caused by inadequate renal perfusion; causes include a significant fall in cardiac output, severe hypotension and intravascular volume depletion, e.g. haemorrhagic or septic shock, peritonitis and pancreatitis. This form of ARF is most commonly seen on the ICU (Bellomo 1997).
- *Postrenal*: caused by obstruction to the flow of urine, e.g. tumour, renal calculi, enlarged prostate; most commonly seen in the community (Feest *et al*. 1993). Although postrenal ARF is rarely encountered in the ICU (Bellomo 1997), obstruction must nevertheless be excluded.
- *Intrinsic*: the most common cause of hospital-acquired ARF; causes include acute tubular necrosis and nephrotoxic drugs.

In all cases, particularly if the patient has persistent anuria or intermittent anuria, it is important to exclude bladder outflow obstruction: this possibility should be suspected in patients who have previously had prostate enlargement or who have had trauma or recent surgery to the pelvic area (Hinds & Watson 1996). In addition, if the patient is catheterised it is important to exclude a blocked catheter.

Diagnosis

The diagnosis of ARF can be confirmed by:

- oliguria on the ICU, this is usually the first sign (Hinds & Watson 1996);

- progressive rise in blood creatinine and urea levels;
- metabolic acidosis;
- hyperkalaemia;
- retention of salt and water.

Once bladder outflow obstruction has been excluded it is important to establish whether the patient is in prerenal, intrarenal or postrenal failure (Hinds & Watson 1996).

Clinical course

The clinical course of ARF can be classified into four distinct phases (Finn 1990).

- *Onset phase*: period of time from the onset of the precipitating event and oliguria.
- *Oliguric/non-oliguric phase*: in the oliguric phase the total urine output is <400 ml in 24 h. The longer this phase continues, the poorer the prognosis for renal recovery (King 1995). The non-oliguric phase can usually be associated with nephrotoxic agents and although urine output may not be reduced, the ability to produce a concentrated urine is severely impaired causing a drop in solute excretion.
- *Diuretic phase*: this is marked by increased urine output, sometimes 3000 ml in 24 h. It is essential to maintain hydration.
- *Recovery phase*.

The prognosis depends on its severity and whether the patient is critically ill.

The mortality rate for patients who have ARF in the presence of multi-organ failure is 60–100% (Lohr *et al.* 1988; Liano *et al.* 1989; and Spiegel *et al.* 1991). However the mortality rate is less than 10% in patients who are not critically ill and who have isolated ARF (Corwin & Bonventre 1989).

Prevention of ARF

Due to the poor prognosis, prevention of ARF in the critically ill patient is paramount. It is important to be able to recognise the early signs of impaired renal function; provided chronic renal failure is prevented, recovery of renal tissue (unlike other major organs) is usually complete (Woodrow 2000). According to Hinds and Watson (1996) the following steps should be taken to try to prevent ARF:

- early identification of those patients at risk;
- careful support of the cardiovascular system (this should include rapid expansion of the circulating volume when indicated);
- judicious use of inotropes when required;
- careful maintenance of crystalloid balance:
- aggressive treatment of sepsis:
- avoidance of nephrotoxic drugs.

Complications of ARF

Hyperkalaemia is the most serious electrolyte imbalance seen in ARF (Bellomo 1997). Characteristic ECG changes include elevated and pointed T waves. Cardiac arrhythmias and cardiac arrest may ensue and active treatment is normally required, e.g. calcium resonium, insulin (and dextrose), renal replacement therapy and in extreme situations intravenous calcium chloride. Continuous cardiac monitoring is essential to ensure early detection of cardiac arrhythmias.

In cases of metabolic acidosis, although active correction is rarely required, if the patient's minute ventilation is markedly increased (resulting from cerebrospinal fluid acidosis) renal replacement therapy is recommended (sodium bicarbonate is no longer advocated (Bellomo 1997)).

A uraemic patient is more susceptible to infection due to impaired leucocyte function, antibody formation and cellular immune responses (Hinds & Watson 1996). Over 70% of patients with ARF develop an infection (McMurray et al. 1978).

Adequate nutritional support is required. A critically ill patient with ARF should receive aggressive, protein-rich nutritional support, either enterally or parenterally; calorie requirements are no different to other ICU patients without ARF (Bellomo *et al.* 1991). Potassium, sodium and fluid intake should be restricted (Smith 1998). Close monitoring of blood glucose levels is essential, particularly if the patient is on dietary supplements.

The patient who is in the oliguric phase of ARF requires careful fluid balance assessment. To prevent volume overload, a general working rule is the previous day's urine output plus 500 ml for insensible loss (Smith 1998). Consideration must be given to such variables as pyrexia, diarrhoea and wound drainage.

Serial weights may be more reliable than fluid balance assessment but are not widely used due to technical difficulties; rapid daily gains and losses in weight are usually related to changes in fluid volume (Smith 1998). It is also important to observe for signs of fluid overload, e.g. raised CVP, generalised oedema, pulmonary oedema and dyspnoea.

Clinical features of uraemia include nausea, vomiting, hiccoughs, confusion, irritability, altered conscious level, infection and bleeding. It is important to observe for these complications and treatment appropriately.

MONITORING DURING RENAL REPLACEMENT THERAPY

The three most common methods of renal replacement therapy are *haemodialysis*, *haemofiltration* (Fig. 5.2) and *peritoneal dialysis*. Whichever method is used, close monitoring during treatment is essential as complications, some of which are life-threatening, may occur. The key aspects of monitoring for each method are described below.

Haemodialysis and haemofiltration

Blood biochemistry, a full blood count and clotting profile are taken as a screening prior to the procedure to provide a baseline. To facilitate patient monitoring pulse oximetry is used.

ECG monitoring is necessary, as cardiac arrhythmias can

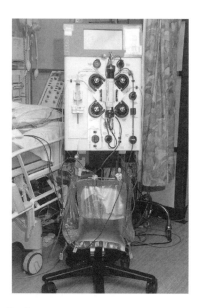

Fig. 5.2 Haemofiltration

occur, particularly if hypokalaemia is present. Hypotension will occur if the rate of fluid being removed in the dialyser exceeds the plasma refilling rate in the patient (Smith 1998), so haemodynamic measurements are also required. In addition during the first 2 h of therapy a sudden drop in blood pressure can occur following fluid drainage (Mallett & Dougherty 2000).

A strict fluid balance must be maintained to prevent accidental hypovolaemia and hypervolaemia, and a careful watch kept on the patient's temperature as circulating the blood outside the body may precipitate hypothermia. Pyrexia may indicate infection.

Circuit pressure monitoring is also important – a rise may indicate clotting of the line. The patient's coagulation status must be closely monitored: anticoagulation of the circuit is often required and the patient is therefore at risk of haemorrhage, so any signs of bleeding from vascular access sites, mucous membranes, GI tract, etc. should be noted. As the blood circulates ensure the bubble trap fluid remains constant.

Complications of haemodialysis and haemofiltration
These include the following.

- *Haemolysis*, resulting from damage to red blood cells as it passes through the pump, can lead to hyperkalaemia and cardiac arrest. Observe for chest pain and dyspnoea. Blood in the venous circuit may have the appearance of 'port wine' (Adam & Osborne 1999).
- *Air embolism*: observe for chest pain and dyspnoea.
- *Reaction to the membrane*: if a cellulose-based cuprophane (dialyser membrane) is used, it may cause a systematic inflammatory response syndrome (Hakim 1993) which can lead to delayed renal recovery and increased mortality (Hakim *et al.* 1994).
- *Disequilibrium*: this is caused by a sudden removal of urea and uraemic toxins and the patient can present with headache, vomiting, restlessness, convulsions and coma (Adam & Osborne 1999).
- *Infection*: strict attention must be paid to maintaining aseptic conditions at all times.

Peritoneal dialysis
Complications of peritoneal dialysis include hyperglycaemia, abdominal fluid leaks, hydrothorax, respiratory embarrassment caused by abdominal distension, significant protein loss from the membrane and mechanical problems with the catheter itself (Bellomo 1997).

Specific monitoring of various parameters of the patient's condition is equally important in this form of renal replacement therapy. The respiratory rate should be watched to ensure that the presence of dialysate in the abdomen does not restrict abdominal movement and cause respiratory embarrassment.

ECG monitoring is again necessary: cardiovascular complications include myocardial infarction and cardiac arrhythmias (Khanna *et al.* 1993). In addition changes in the heart rate may be indicative of shock or overhydration.

As regards haemodynamic measurements, cycle times together with volumes of dialysate should be closely monitored; hypotension can occur if fluid removal is too great or too rapid. Circulating volume should be regularly assessed. Diffusion of glucose from the dialysate into the body can lead to hypoglycaemia, so blood glucose measurements must be taken.

Measure inflow of the dialysate and observe for abdominal pain which may indicate too much dialysate per cycle or peritonitis.

Dialysate outflow failure is one of the most common operational problems associated with PD. The dialysate fluid should be at least equal to the volume of fluid infused; factors causing outflow problems include a kinked catheter, decreased bowel motility, obstruction by fibrin plugs or strands and peritonitis (Adam & Osborne 1999).

Strict fluid balance must again be maintained to prevent accidental hypovolaemia and hypervolaemia.

Signs of infection to watch for include peritonitis (cloudy dialysate, abdominal pain and tenderness, pyrexia) so culture the returned dialysate on a daily basis. The presence of erythema and purulent exudate at the catheter exit site indicates exit site infection (Luzar 1991): its incidence can be reduced by securely anchoring the catheter to the patient's skin (Gokal *et al.* 1993). Regular monitoring of the patient's temperature is essential.

Finally, dialysis fluid may leak around the exit site so this should be closely watched for.

Scenario

Mr Yates was admitted to the ICU after a blunt abdominal injury sustained in an industrial accident. He was ventilated following a diagnostic laparotomy and repair of mesenteric tear. He was progressing steadily over the next 24 h when his condition deteriorated. He became cardiovascularly unstable and required inotropic support. He was hyperpyrexial with a white cell blood count of 27.8. Intra-abdominal sepsis was suspected.

He was taken to theatre for a further laparotomy to ascertain the focus. At operation haemorrhagic pancreatitis was diagnosed and several irrigation drains were inserted into the abdomen and saline irrigation commenced. After return to the unit his condition deteriorated with inotropic requirements increasing and oliguria developing. How would you manage oliguria?

It is important to ensure that the urinary catheter is not blocked or kinked. Diuretics were administered without effect and anuria developed. The patient's blood chemistry was:

Potassium: 6.8 mmol/l

Serum urea: 24 mmoml/s

Creatinine: 420

A diagnosis of acute tubular necrosis (ATN) was made. What would you do now?

Haemofiltration was established without complications, removing 120 ml/h, using heparin as the anticoagulant in the circuit. Blood was taken for APTT levels until this was within therapeutic range to prevent the filter clotting. Initially blood was taken twice daily for biochemical analysis to ascertain the efficacy of haemofiltration in terms of reducing the serum creatinine and urea and maintaining a stable serum potassium.

Haemofiltration continued for a further 10 days during which time sepsis abated and renal function returned to normal. The patient made a full recovery from this episode of ATN secondary to sepsis.

CONCLUSION

Monitoring renal function is central to the care of a critically ill patient. It can provide an indication to the function of the kidneys as well as the performance of other major systems of the body. The early recognition and prompt treatment of acute renal failure is essential if prognosis is to be maximised.

REFERENCES

Adam, S. & Osborne, S. (1999) *Critical Care Nursing: Science and Practice*. Oxford Medical Publications, Oxford.

Bellomo, R. (1997) Acute renal failure. In: T.E. Oh, ed. *Intensive Care Manual*, 4th edn. Butterworth Heinemann, Oxford.

Bellomo, R., Martin, H., Parkin, G. *et al.* (1991) Continuous arteriovenous hemodiafiltration in the critically ill: influence on major nutrient balances. *Intensive Care Medicine* **17**, 399–402.

Cook, R. (1996) Urinalysis: ensuring accurate urine testing. *Nursing Standard* **10** (46), 49–52.

Corwin, H.L. & Bonventre, J.V. (1989) Factors influencing survival in acute renal failure. *Semin Di* **2**, 220–225.

Feest, T.G., Round, A. & Hamad, S. (1993) Incidence of severe acute renal failure in adults: results from a community based study. *British Medical Journal* **306**, 481–483.

Finn, W. F. (1990) Diagnosis and management of acute tubular necrosis. *Medical Clinics of North America* **74** (4).

Gokal, R., Ash, S., Holfrich, B. *et al.* (1993) Peritoneal catheters and exit site practices: toward optimum peritoneal access. *Peritoneal Dialysis International* **13**, 29–39.

Gomersall, C. & Oh, T. (1997) Haemodynamic monitoring. In: T. Oh, ed. *Intensive Care Manual*, 4th edn. Butterworth Heinemann, Oxford.

Gosling, P. (1999) Fluid balance in the critically ill: the sodium and water audit. *Care of the Critically Ill* **15** (1), 11–18.

Hakim, R. (1993) Clinical implications of hemodialysis membrane biocompatability. *Kidney International* **44**, 484–494.

Hakim, R., Wingard, R. & Parker, R. (1994) Effect of dialysis membrane in the treatment of patients with acute renal failure. *New England Journal of Medicine* **331**, 1338–1342.

Hamilton, M. (1999) Cause and effects of renal failure. *Nursing Times* **95** (12), 59–60.

Hinds, C.J. & Watson, D. (1996) *Intensive Care: A concise textbook*, 2nd edn. W. B. Saunders, London.

Khanna, R., Nolph, K. & Oreopoulos, D., eds (1993) Complications during peritoneal dialysis. In: *The Essentials of Peritoneal Dialysis*. Kluwer Academic, Dordrecht.

King, B. (1995) Acute renal failure. *Registered Nurse* March, 35–39.

Liano, F., Garcia-Martin, F., Gallego, A. *et al.* (1989) Easy and early prognosis in acute tubular necrosis: a forward of analysis of 228 cases. *Nephron* **51**, 307–313.

Lohr, J.W., McFarlane, M.J. & Grantham, A.J. (1988) A clinical index to predict survival in acute renal failure patients requiring dialysis. *American Journal of Kidney Disease* **11**, 254–259.

Luzar, M. (1991) Exit site infection in CAPD: a review. *Peritoneal Dialysis International* **11**, 333–340.

Mallett, J. & Dougherty, L., eds (2000) *The Royal Marsden Hospital Manual of Clinical Nursing Procedures*. Blackwell Science, Oxford.

McMurray, S.D., Luft, F.C., Maxwell, D.R. *et al.* (1978) Prevailing patterns and predictor variables in patients with acute tubular necrosis. *Archives of Internal Medicine* **138**, 950–955.

Sheppard, M. (2000) Monitoring fluid balance in acutely ill patients. *Nursing Times* **96** (21), 39–40.

Sheppard, M. & Wright, M. (2000) *High Dependency Nursing*, 1st edn, p. 249. Baillière Tindall, London.

Sladen, R.N. (1994) Renal physiology. In: R.D. Miller, E.D. Cucchiara, E. Miller *et al.*, eds. *Anaesthesia*, 4th edn. Churchill Livingstone, New York.

Smith, T. (1998) *Renal Nursing*. Ballière Tindall, London.

Spiegel, D.M., Ullian, M.E., Zerbe, G.O. & Berl, T. (1991) Determinants of survival and recovery in acute renal failure patients dialysed in intensive care units. *American Journal of Nephrology* **11**, 44–47.

Talley, N.J. & O'Connor, S. (1998) *Pocket Clinical Examination*. Blackwell Science, Oxford.

Torrance, C. (1998) Urine testing 1: observation. *Nursing Times* **94** (4), suppl.

Torrance, C. & Elley, K. (1997) Respiration, technique and observation 1. *Nursing Times* **93** (43), Suppl. 1–2.

Toto, K.H. (1992) Acute renal failure: a question of location. *American Journal of Nursing* November, 44–53.

Woodrow, P. (2000) *Intensive Care Nursing, A Framework for Practice*. Routledge, London.

Monitoring Gastrointestinal Function

INTRODUCTION

The importance of the gastrointestinal (GI) tract as a defence system and as an essential resource for other organs is increasingly being recognised. The support of its functions is now considered an essential part of the global treatment of a critically ill patient (Adam & Osborne 1999). It is therefore essential to be able to monitor GI function accurately.

The aim of this chapter is to understand the principles of monitoring GI function.

LEARNING OBJECTIVES

At the end of the chapter the reader will be able to:

❏ describe the assessment of *bowel function*;
❏ discuss the significance of *nausea and vomiting*;
❏ discuss the monitoring of *stomas and fistulas*;
❏ outline the causes of acute *upper gastrointestinal bleeding*;
❏ outline the assessment of *intestinal obstruction*;
❏ discuss the principles of monitoring *pancreatic function*.

ASSESSMENT OF BOWEL FUNCTION

Assessing bowel function can provide important information that can assist in diagnosis and can help in the monitoring of a patient's clinical condition. The following should be noted:

- *patient's normal bowel activity*: frequency of bowel movement and any unexplained changes in bowel habit;
- *consistency of the faeces*: hard, bulky or pellet-like suggestive of constipation; loose, watery and frequent faeces are suggestive of diarrhoea;

- *colour of faeces*: normal faeces should be brown due to the presence of modified bowel pigments (Bruce & Finley 1997); dark faeces can be caused by iron tablets, upper GI haemorrhage causes malena (black tarry faeces);
- *presence of fresh blood* is suggestive of bleeding from the lower bowel, rectum or haemorrhoids;
- *presence of mucous*: normally associated with inflammatory bowel disease;
- *odour*: constipation, malabsorption, diet and bowel infection can cause an offensive odour (pale faeces together with an offensive odour may be suggestive of gall bladder related problems);
- *steatorrhoea*: pale, bulky and offensive stools is a sign of malabsorption of fat;
- *pain on defecation*: possible causes include constipation, haemorrhoids and perianal Crohn's disease;
- *volume of faeces*: particularly if the patient is having diarrhoea.

Adapted from Winney 1998

Constipation

Constipation is a subjective and variable symptom and can be considered as a deviation from the individual's normal bowel function in the presence of additional factors such as straining and discomfort (Taylor 1988). In critically ill patients there are many predisposing factors including enforced bed rest, change in diet, dehydration, medications such as opiates and lack of privacy.

A rectal examination should be undertaken to determine the presence, consistency and volume of faeces in the rectum. It is important to monitor bowel function in order to prevent/relieve constipation.

Diarrhoea

Acute diarrhoea is often short-lived and requires little treatment with the aim of management focusing on resolving symptoms and preventing complications (Taylor 1988). However if the patient develops diarrhoea it is important to ascertain the cause, such as infection, medications, e.g. antibiotics, enteral nutrition. A sample should be sent for MC & S. A stool chart should be maintained and the patient's hydration and nutrition status should be monitored. Regular monitoring of temperature should be undertaken in case there is a gut infection.

Significance of nausea and vomiting

There are many causes of nausea and vomiting (Table 6.1). Acute symptoms can be caused by gastrointestinal tract infections or obstruction of the small bowel; when the symptoms are chronic, pregnancy and drugs should be ruled out as possible causes (Talley & O'Connor 1998). Women are three more times more likely to experience nausea and vomiting than men in the postoperative period (Thompson 1992), particularly during menstruation (Hawthorn 1995).

In all cases of nausea and vomiting the following are important:

- the patient's medical history and present condition;
- examination of the patient's abdomen to determine whether there is pain, tenderness, guarding, presence of bowel sounds;
- the patient's medication regime, both past and current;
- blood biochemical assessment;
- a rectal examination;
- a plain abdominal X-ray.

Bruce & Finley 1997

The timing of vomiting together with the volume and consistency of the vomit are also helpful.

Timing of vomiting

Vomiting that occurs more than an hour after eating is characteristic of obstruction of the gastric outlet, while early

Table **6.1** Causes of nausea and vomiting

Intestinal obstructions	Adhesions; intussusception of bowel; change in intraluminal pressure due to presence of malignant tumour or ulcer pyloric stenosis
Inflammatory processes	Gastroenteritis; peritonitis; acute pancreatitis; acute cholecystitis
Motility disorders	Pyloric stenosis; postoperative illness; constipation
Irritations	Bacterial or viral infection; bacterial toxins in food poisoning; gastric manipulation during surgery/ investigations
Drug treatments	Chemotherapy; opiate analgesics; many antibiotics
Psychic/neurological factors	Raised intercranial pressure; severe pain; unpleasant odours;offensive sights
Metabolic imbalance	Diabetic ketoacidosis; uraemia from renal disease
Miscellaneous	Disease of the ear, e.g. tinnitus or Ménière's disease; migraine; motion sickness; pregnancy

Adapted and reproduced by permission of Churchill Livingstone from Bruce & Finlay 1997

morning vomiting is typical of pregnancy, alcoholism and raised intracranial pressure (Talley & O'Connor 1998).

Volume of vomit

The volume of the vomit is important: a large volume may be indicative of gastric outflow obstruction. If there are small amounts of vomit it is important to ensure that the patient is actually vomiting and not just expectorating – the litmus paper test is recommended.

Consistency of vomit

The consistency is important:

- *'coffee-grounds'*: old blood clots in vomit; can also be caused by iron tablets, red wine and of course coffee ingestion;
- *fresh blood*: the presence of fresh blood is indicative of bleeding from the upper gastrointestinal tract
- *yellow/green*: presence of bile and upper small bowel contents is suggestive of obstruction;
- *faeculent*: brown offensive material from the small bowel, a late sign of small intestinal obstruction (Talley & O'Connor 1998);
- *projectile*: causes include pyloric stenosis and raised intracranial pressure.

MONITORING STOMAS AND FISTULAS

Stomas

Several factors can influence the characteristics of output from stomas including medication, diet and amount of bowel removed. The position of the stoma is also significant: basically the more proximal the stoma, the more fluid the effluent and the more caustic its effect on the skin due to the presence of proteolytic enzymes (Meadows 1997). The skin surrounding the stoma should be closely observed for early signs of maceration (Myers 1998). Documentation of the size, length and colour should be regularly undertaken and output from the stoma should be recorded.

Fistulas

An enterocutaneaous fistula (abnormal communication between a section of the gastrointestinal tract and the skin) can lead to a life-threatening deterioration in the patient's condition with sepsis, electrolyte disturbances, malnutrition and dehydration (Rinsema 1994). Most enterocutaneous fistulas occur following surgery; monitoring priorities include recording the consistency and volume of the effluent and observing the surrounding skin for maceration.

ACUTE UPPER GASTROINTESTINAL BLEEDING

Acute upper gastrointestinal bleeding accounts for over 28 000 admissions in the UK each year and carries a 10% mortality rate (Morris 1992). Common causes include duodenal and gastric ulceration, gastritis, Mallory–Weiss tear and oesophageal varices.

The vomit may either be bright red or coffee-ground in appearance, depending on the length of time the blood has been in contact with gastric secretions (gastric acid converts bright red haemoglobin to brown hematin) and on the amount of gastric contents at the time of the bleeding (Hudak *et al.* 1998).

Although most GI bleeds stop spontaneously, approximately 20% will rebleed in hospital and many of these will need surgical intervention.

Monitoring priorities include:

- assessing for signs of hypovolaemia and shock;
- estimating blood loss and accurate maintenance of fluid balance;
- determining the cause of the bleed if possible (Table 6.2);
- monitoring fluid balance;
- monitoring the function of other major systems;
- laboratory investigations, e.g. FBC, prothrombin time, liver function tests, platelet count, urea and electrolytes.

If the patient requires a Sengstaken tube, as is sometimes the case in bleeding oesophageal varices, close monitoring of tube position together with the patient's airway and respiratory status is important.

ASSESSMENT OF INTESTINAL OBSTRUCTION

Intestinal obstruction can occur in either the small or large

Table 6.2 Causes of upper gastrointestinal bleeding

Common	Duodenal and gastric ulceration; oesophagitis; gastritis; duodenitis; varices; Mallory–Weiss tear
Less common	Carcinomas; bleeding diathesis; leiomyomas; aortic aneurysm fistula
Rare (less than 1%)	Dieulafoy lesion; angiomas; hereditary haemorrahagic telangiectasia; pseudoxanthoma elasticum; Ehlers–Danlos syndrome; haemobilia; pancreatic bleeding; foreign body

Reproduced by permission of Churchill Livingstone from Bruce & Finlay 1997

bowel. It can lead to bowel strangulation, infarction, and perforation resulting in potentially life-threatening peritoneal and systemic infection (Hudak *et al*. 1998). It can be classified as mechanical or non-mechanical.

Mechanical obstruction results from a physical blockage of the intestinal lumen which may be complete or incomplete. Causes include adhesions, malignancy, hernias, bolus obstruction and bowel strangulation, e.g. volvulus. Non-mechanical obstruction is caused by ineffective intestinal peristalsis (paralytic ileus), causes of which include trauma, handling of the bowel during surgery, peritonitis and electrolyte imbalance (Hudak *et al*. 1998).

Detailed below are the key monitoring considerations:

- *blood pressure* and *pulse measurements* to detect early signs of shock;
- *temperature* – pyrexia is usually present, though does not normally exceed 37.8°C (Hudak *et al*. 1998);
- *abdominal girth measurements*: abdominal distension is a key clinical feature;
- *vomiting*: the higher the obstruction, the more profuse the vomit;
- *fluid and electrolyte balance*;

- *abdominal pain*: characteristics and severity;
- *bowel function*: consistency of faeces, regularity, volume.

PRINCIPLES OF MONITORING PANCREATIC FUNCTION

The pancreas secretes water to dilute chyme, bicarbonate to neutralise postgastric chyme and enzymes to help with digestion. Its endocrine function is discussed in Chapter 8.

Acute pancreatitis, which is associated with significant morbidity and mortality rates (Steinberg & Tenner 1994), is commonly caused by long-term alcohol abuse and gallbladder disease, which account for over 75% of cases (Adam & Osborne 1999). Pancreatitis can compromise most of the major systems in the body. Therefore close monitoring is required. The key priorities are listed below.

- *Haemodynamic monitoring*: hypovolaemia and fluid volume imbalances may be present (large volumes of fluid can leak into extravascular spaces).
- *Pulse oximetry and arterial blood gas analysis*: respiratory failure can be a complication.
- *ECG monitoring*: electrolyte imbalances can cause arrhythmias.
- *Blood sugar estimations*: hyperglycaemia may occur as a result of impaired insulin production and increased release of glucagon.
- *Temperature*: the main cause of pyrexia is hypermetabolism, though infection may also be the cause (Woodrow 2000).
- *Nutrition status*: patient will be nil by mouth, parenteral nutrition will probably be started (Robin *et al.* 1990). If there is long-term alcohol abuse, nutrition is an even greater priority.
- *Serum amylase*: usually increases up to tenfold within 6 h (Reece-Smith 1997).
- *Pain*: the patient may have severe abdominal pain.

Scenario

Mr White, a 48-year-old man, was admitted to the medical ward with a history of haemetemesis. He was fully conscious, looked pale, had cool peripheries and there was fresh blood around his mouth. Oxygen was commenced. What would your monitoring priorities initially be?

The patient's vital signs were taken: BP 80/50, pulse 120/min and thready, resps 30/min. and SpO_2 was difficult to obtain. What do these measurements tell you?

An initial diagnosis was made: hypovolaemic shock secondary to heametemesis. IV access was established with two wide bore cannulas, one in each arm. Bloods were taken for LFTs, U+Es, FBC, X match for 6 units + 2 units FFP, clotting screen and fluid resuscitation was commenced with Hartmann's solution STAT. Intravenous Omeprazole was administered. A urinary catheter and central venous catheter were inserted. Arterial blood gas results were within normal limits.

What monitoring would you now do?

The CVP reading is: 1 mmHg. BP is now 70/50, HR 130, resps 30 and the patient is becoming disorientated. Urine output is minimal and a blocked catheter is ruled out. SpO_2 is still unobtainable. What do these measurements tell you?

The patient's hypovolaemia appears to be deteriorating despite fluid resuscitation. The CVP reading is low, though caution is required as it is an isolated reading (serial readings are more helpful). The patient's conscious level continued to deteriorate, together with his vital signs. The patient required urgent transfusion and review by surgical team. Following an urgent gastroscopy, the patient was transferred to theatre for oversewing of a bleeding gastric ulcer.

CONCLUSION

Monitoring GI function is central to the management of a critically ill patient. The principles of monitoring have been discussed and include assessment of bowel action, the significance of nausea and vomiting and key aspects of monitoring for intestinal obstruction and pancreatitis.

REFERENCES

Adam, S. & Osborne, S. (1999) *Critical Care Nursing: Science and Practice*. Oxford Medical Publications, Oxford.

Bruce, L. & Finley, T.M.D. (1997) *Nursing in Gastroenterology*. Churchill Livingstone, London.

Hawthorn, J. (1995) *Understanding and Management of Nausea and Vomiting*. Blackwell Scientific Publications, Oxford.

Hudak, C.M., Gallo, B.M. & Morton, P.G. (1998) *Critical Care Nursing a Holistic Approach*, 7th edn. Lippincott, New York.

Johnson, C. (1998) Severe acute pancreatitis: a continuing challenge for the intensive care team. *British Journal of Intensive Care* **8** (4), 130–137.

Kennedy, J. (1997) Enteral feeding for the critically ill patient. *Nursing Standard* **11** (33), 39–43.

Mallett, J. & Dougherty, L. (2000) eds. *The Royal Marsden Hospital Manual of Clinical Nursing Procedures*. Blackwell Science, Oxford.

Meadows, C. (1997) Stoma and fistula care. In: L. Bruce & T.M.D. Finley, eds *Nursing in Gastroenterology*. Churchill Livingstone, London.

Morris, A. (1992) Upper gastrointestinal haemorrhage – endoscopic approaches to diagnosis and treatment. In I. Gilmore & R. Shields, eds *Gastrointestinal Emergencies*. W.B. Saunders, London.

Myers, A. (1998) Inside stories. *Nursing Times* **94** (20), 66–67.

Reece-Smith, H. (1997) Pancreatitis. *Care of the Critically Ill* **13** (4), 135–138.

Rinsema, W. (1994) Gastrointestinal fistula: management and results of treatment. Datawyse, Maastricht.

Robin, A., Campbell, R. & Palani, C. (1990) Total parenteral nutrition during acute pancreatitis: clinical experience with 156 patients. *World Journal of Surgery* **14**, 572–579.

Steinberg, W. & Tenner, S. (1994) Acute pancreatitis. *New England Journal of Medicine* **330**, 1198–1210.

Talley, N.J. & O'Connor, S. (1998) *Pocket Clinical Examination*. Blackwell Science, Oxford.

Taylor, S. (1988) A guide to nasogastric feeding equipment. *Professional Nurse* **4**, 91–94.

Thompson, H.J. (1992) Post-operative nausea and vomiting. *British Journal of Theatre Nursing* **29** (5), 1130.

Winney, J. (1998) Constipation. *Nursing Standard* **13** (11), 49–56.

Woodrow, P. (2000) *Intensive Care Nursing. A Framework for Practice*. Routledge, London.

7

Monitoring Hepatic Function

INTRODUCTION

Patients admitted to an ICU with a primarily non-hepatic disease frequently develop hepatic dysfunction (Hawker 1997). If acute liver failure (ALF) develops widespread hepatocyte necrosis can lead to severely impaired hepatic function and encephalopathy. Although recovery from ALF on the ICU is usually good (Wiles 1999), overall survival is only 20–25% on medical therapy alone, with 70% requiring transplantation (Hawker 1997).

The liver, the largest organ in the body, has three broad functions: *synthesis*, *storage* and *detoxification*. Any hepatic dysfunction can affect most of the other major systems in the body. Patients with ALF frequently develop multiorgan failure and associated complications include encephalopathy, systemic infections, cerebral oedema, haemodynamic instability, coagulopathy, and renal and metabolic dysfunction (Herrera 1998). Close monitoring of hepatic function and complications of ALF is paramount; prevention or timely recognition and management of these complications is crucial (Shoemaker *et al.* 1995).

The aim of this chapter is to understand the principles of monitoring hepatic function, with specific reference to the complications of ALF.

LEARNING OBJECTIVES

At the end of the chapter the reader will be able to:

❏ outline the *functions* of the liver;
❏ list the causes of *liver dysfunction and ALF*;

❑ discuss the *clinical features of ALF*;
❑ discuss how to monitor the specific *complications of ALF*.

FUNCTIONS OF THE LIVER

The clinical features of ALF are largely attributable to the failure of normal hepatic functions (Hinds & Watson 1996). Therefore in order to appreciate the principles of monitoring hepatic function, it is essential to understand the functions of the liver, which include:

- metabolism of carbohydrates, fat, protein and bilirubin;
- storage of vitamins and minerals;
- detoxification of both internal and external substances;
- formation and storage of glycogen;
- production and storage of clotting factors prothrombin and vitamin K;
- formation of amino acids and proteins, e.g. albumin;
- production of heat;
- manufacture and secretion of bile.

Wilson & Waugh 1996

CAUSES OF LIVER DYSFUNCTION AND ALF

Causes of liver dysfunction include:

- *hypoperfusion*, the commonest cause (Hickman & Potter 1990 and Woodrow 2000);
- *drugs*;
- *fatty infiltration of the liver* precipitated by high calorie parenteral nutrition and benign post operative cholestasis (Hinds & Watson 1996);
- *multiple organ failure.*

Causes of ALF include:

- *paracetamol overdose*: the commonest cause in the UK (Langley & Pain 1994 and Stanley *et al.* 1995);
- *drugs*;

- *alcohol, industrial solvents, mushrooms* (Sussman 1996);
- *hepatitis* and other viruses.

CLINICAL FEATURES OF ALF

A patient with ALF will have clinical manifestations that are directly related to the degree of impaired hepatic function (Budden & Vink 1996). Early clinical features include nausea, vomiting, anorexia, abdominal pain, flatulence, diarrhoea, steatorrhoea, pyrexia, pruritus, jaundice, loss of weight and dark urine (Ignatavicius & Bayne 1991).

Jaundice, a yellow pigmentation of the tissues, may be observed in the skin and conjunctiva and is a sign of abnormal bilirubin metabolism and excretion. Although the normal serum bilirubin is 3–13 mmol/l, jaundice may not be evident until the level has risen to 34 mmol/l (Wilson & Waugh 1996) (other causes of jaundice include haemolysis and obstruction to the flow of bile).

Liver function tests should be performed at least daily. A plasma bilirubin concentration of >300 mmol/l is a poor prognostic sign (Hawker 1997). INR is a useful indicator of hepatic function.

MONITORING THE SPECIFIC COMPLICATIONS OF ALF

Encephalopathy

Encephalopathy is a characteristic clinical feature of ALF. The exact cause is unknown, though it is possible that the accumulation of circulating toxic substances plays a key role. It is important to recognise the early signs of encephalopathy, thus allowing early treatment (Budden & Vink 1996).

It can be classified into four grades depending on severity (Table 7.1) and usually progresses over several days, though deep coma can develop in just a few hours (Hinds & Watson 1996). Although it is important to document the grade of encephalopathy, repeated clinical examination is more helpful

Table 7.1 Grading of hepatic encephalopathy

Grade 0:	Normal mental state
Grade 1:	Changes in mental state, e.g. lack of awareness, anxiety, euphoria, reduced attention span, difficulty with adding and subtracting
Grade 2:	Lethargy, disorientation (for time), personality changes, inappropriate behaviour
Grade 3:	Stupor, but responsive to stimuli; gross disorientation, confusion
Grade 4:	Coma

Reproduced by permission of MacLennan T. Petty from material reproduced in Talley & O'Connor 2001

Table 7.2 Clinical examination of encephalopathy

Grade of encephalopathy	Tone and reflexes	Response to pain	Pupils
GRADE 1	Normal		
GRADE 2	Brisk reflexes and increased tone	Obeys	Normal
GRADE 3	Up-going plantar reflexes, clonus	Localises, flexes hippus	'Hyper-reactive'
GRADE 4	Sustained clonus	Extends	Dilated, sluggish
BRAIN DEATH	Flaccid, absent reflexes	None	Fixed and dilated

Reproduced by permission of Butterworth-Heinemann from Oh 1997

if the clinical course is to be more accurately followed (Hawker 1997) (Table. 7.2).

The neurological status of the patient should be evaluated and closely monitored; in brief, the conscious level, motor movement, sensory pupil size and reaction to light should be examined. In advanced encephalopathy the pupils may become dilated and react sluggishly to light; if they become dilated and unreactive brainstem coning is likely (Hawker 1997).

Orientation should be monitored together with concentration span, restlessness, personality and behaviour changes, emotional lability, drowsiness, slurred or slow speech and disturbances in the sleep pattern. A generalised increase in muscle tone is an early sign of progression of encephalopathy. Spontaneous hyperventilation is common which can result in a significant alkalosis (Hawker 1997). The respiratory rate should therefore be regularly recorded together with blood gas analysis.

Sedatives, often administered to these patients, can cause a rapid deterioration of mental status and are therefore not recommended (Shoemaker *et al.* 1995). The degree of electroencephalographic (EEG) changes correlate with the degree of cerebral dysfunction; serial EEGs together with clinical assessment can be performed to determine the patient's progress (Hinds & Watson 1996).

Cerebral oedema

Cerebral oedema is the leading cause of death in patients with ALF (Plevris *et al.* 1998), being present in over 80% of grade IV encephalopathy (Hawker 1997). The clinical signs of cerebral oedema, i.e. systemic hypertension, decerebrate posturing and abnormal pupillary reflexes are generally attributed to brainstem compression. Cerebral oedema provokes intracranial hypertension that impairs cerebral perfusion pressure.

Cerebral blood flow correlates to arterial pressure and not cardiac output in patients with ALF; strict cardiovascular control is important when pressure-passive cerebral circulation is present in order to maintain continuous and adequate cerebral oxygenation and avoid the development of cerebral hyperaemia and cerebral oedema (Larsen *et al.* 2000). Close cardiac and haemodynamic monitoring is therefore imperative.

Intracranial pressure (ICP) monitoring allows the early

detection and treatment of cerebral oedema (Lockhart-Wood 1996). Although it is a well-established treatment, complications (Waite 1993), which are sometimes fatal (Blei *et al*. 1993), can occur. For each patient, the risk–benefit ratio should be considered, particularly as positive outcomes have been achieved without ICP monitoring (Sheil *et al*. 1991).

Coagulopathy and haemorrhaging

Patients with ALF frequently develop severe coagulopathy; the hepatic synthesis of clotting factors is impaired and as a result the clotting times, e.g. INR, PTT, are always prolonged. In addition qualitative and quantitative defects of platelets occur (O'Grady & Williams 1986). The INR, the most useful test for monitoring the relative synthesis of coagulation factors during the course of hepatic failure (Shoemaker *et al*. 1995), is a useful prognostic indicator (Hawker 1997).

The most common site for haemorrhage is the gastrointestinal tract (Hawker 1997); other sites include the nasopharynx, respiratory tract and skin puncture sites (Hawker 1997). It is important to monitor for signs of haemorrhage, e.g. in faeces, urine, skin, sputum, endotracheal tube and vomit.

Renal failure

Renal failure is a common complication of ALF (Hinds & Watson 1996), occurring in approximately 75% of patients with grade IV encephalopathy following paracetamol overdose and in <30% of other aetiologies (O'Grady & Williams 1986). Common clinical manifestations include oliguria, increased plasma concentrations of creatinine, low sodium content in the urine and previous normal renal function (Hawker 1997). Urine output should therefore be closely monitored.

Sepsis

Bacterial infection is common, occurring in 80% of patients with ALF (Rolando *et al*. 1990). Sepsis worsens hepatic function (Rolando *et al*. 1990). Septic patients are more likely to develop renal failure and gastrointestinal haemorrhaging and have a significantly higher mortality risk than non-septic patients (Shoemaker *et al.* 1995).

The patient's vital signs should be closely monitored, though pyrexia and an increased white cell count are absent in 30% of patents with documented bacterial infection (Hawker 1997). As pulmonary and urinary tract infections are the most common (Shoemaker *et al.* 1995), sputum and urine should be scrutinised and samples sent for microbiology, culture and sensitivity. Although ascites may be associated with ALF, spontaneous bacterial peritonitis is a rare complication (Poddar *et al.* 1998).

Metabolic disturbances

Hypoglycaemia is common, resulting from impaired gluconeogenesis, reduced glycogen stores and increased circulating levels of insulin (Hawker 1997). Blood glucose levels should be measured regularly. Primary respiratory alkalosis is common in spontaneously breathing patients (see the section on Encephalopathy earlier). Impaired hepatic synthesis of urea and hypokalaemia can cause metabolic alkalosis. Electrolyte disturbances are very common.

Scenario

Mrs Jones was admitted to the medical HDU with a diagnosis of acute on chronic liver failure. On admission her condition was stable with normal haemodynamic parameters. She was, however, graded at level 1 hepatic encephalopathy, alteration to her mood and slight confusion. She had obvious abdominal ascites and pitting ankle oedema. Bloods were taken for analysis: LFTs, U & Es, clotting time, FBC. What are her monitoring priorities?

Her airway was monitored and she had supplementary O_2 at 35% via a humidifier. Continuous SpO_2 monitoring was instigated and continuous ECG along with hourly fluid balance. Regular assessment of conscious level was performed to detect

---

any early deterioration, which is possible in these patients with encephalopathy. Blood glucose levels were monitored hourly initially, as the liver's function of gluconeogenesis is reduced and hypoglycaemia is common in such patients.

A low protein high carbohydrate enteral feed was commenced after ensuring that there was no active bleeding in the GI tract. Careful monitoring of the patient was performed to ascertain if active bleeding had occurred as clotting disorders are a common occurrence in liver failure due to the storage of clotting factors in the liver. After several days of careful monitoring and support Mrs Jones's conscious state began to improve and she was transferred to the general ward for further support.

CONCLUSION

ICU patients frequently develop hepatic dysfunction. If ALF develops widespread hepatocyte necrosis can lead to severely impaired hepatic function and life-threatening complications may result. Close monitoring of hepatic function and complications of ALF is paramount if the patient's prognosis is to improve.

REFERENCES

Blei, A., Olafsson, S., Webster, S. & Levy, R. (1993) Complications of intracranial pressure monitoring in fulminant hepatic failure. *The Lancet* **341**, 157–158.

Budden, L. & Vink, R. (1996) Paracetamol overdose: pathophysiology and nursing management. *British Journal of Nursing* **5** (3), 145–152.

Hawker, F. (1997) Hepatic failure. In T. Oh, ed. *Intensive Care Manual*, 4th edn. Butterworth Heinemann, Oxford.

Herrera, J. (1998) Management of acute liver failure. *Digestive Diseases* **16** (5), 274–283.

Hickman, P. & Potter, J. (1990) Mortality associated with ischaemic hepatitis. *Australian and New Zealand Journal of Medicine* **20**, 32–34.

Hinds, C.J. & Watson, D. (1996) *Intensive Care: a concise textbook*, 2nd edn. W.B. Saunders, London.

Ignatavicius, D. & Bayne, M. (1991) *Medical-Surgical: A Nursing Process Approach*. W.B. Saunders, Philadelphia.

Langley, S. & Pain, J. (1994) Surgery and liver dysfunction. *Care of the Critically Ill* **10** (3), 113–117.

Larsen, F., Strauss, G., Knudsen, G. *et al.* (2000) Cerebral perfusion, cardiac output and arterial pressure in patients with fulminant hepatic failure. *Critical Care Medicine* **28** (4), 996–1000.

Lockhart-Wood, K. (1996) Developments in practice. Cerebral oedema in fulminant hepatic failure. *Nursing in Critical Care* **1** (6), 283–285.

Mallett, J. & Dougherty, L. (2000) eds *The Royal Marsden Hospital Manual of Clinical Nursing Procedures.* Blackwell Science, Oxford.

O'Grady, J.G. & Williams, R. (1986) Management of acute liver failure. *Schweizerische Medizidinische Wochenschrift* **116** (17), 541–544.

Oh, T. (ed.) (1997) *Intensive Care Manual*, 4th edn. Butterworth-Heinemann, Oxford.

Plevris, J., Schina, M. & Hayes, P. (1998) Review article: the management of acute liver failure. *Alimentary Pharmacology and Therapeutics* **12** (5), 405–418.

Poddar, U., Chawla, Y., Dhiman, R. *et al.* (1998) Spontaneous bacterial peritonitis in fulminant hepatic failure. *Journal of Gastroenterology and Hepatology* **13** (1), 109–111.

Rolando, P.G., Harvey, F., Brahm, J. *et al.* (1990) Prospective study of bacterial infection in acute liver failure: an analysis of fifty patients. *Hepatology* **11**, 49–53.

Sheil, A., McCaughan, G., Isai, H. *et al.* (1991) Acute and subacute fulminant hepatic failure: the role of liver transplantation. *Medical Journal of Australia* **154**, 724–728.

Shoemaker, W., Ayres, S., Grenuik, A. & Hollrook, P. (1995) *Textbook of Critical Care.* W.B. Saunders, London.

Stanley, A., Lee, A. & Hayes, P. (1995) Management of acute liver failure. *British Journal of Intensive Care* **5** (1), 8–15.

Sussman, N. (1996) Fulminant hepatic failure. In: D. Zakim & T. Boyer eds, *Hepatology: A Textbook of Liver Disease* 3rd edn. W.B. Saunders, Philadelphia.

Talley, N. & O'Connor, S. (2001) *Clinical Examination*, 4th edn. MacLennan + Petty, East Gardens, NSW, Australia.

Waite, L. (1993) Commentary on complications of intracranial pressure monitoring in fulminant hepatic failure. *AACN Nursing Scan in Critical Care* **3** (6), 19–20.

Wiles, C. (1999) Critical care apheresis: hepatic failure. *Therapeutic Apheresis* **3** (1), 31–33.

Wilson, K. & Waugh, A. (1996) *Anatomy and Physiology in Health and Illness* 8th edn. Churchill Livingstone, London.

Woodrow, P. (2000) *Intensive Care Nursing, A Framework for Practice.* Routledge, London.

Monitoring Endocrine Function

8

INTRODUCTION

Monitoring endocrine function is an important aspect of caring for the critically ill patient. Disorders of this function can be life-threatening and early detection of problems through close monitoring is essential.

For the purpose of this chapter, only the potentially life-threatening disorders of endocrine function will be discussed. An understanding of the physiology of the endocrine system is important if the effects of its malfunction are to be appreciated.

The aim of this chapter is to understand the principles of monitoring endocrine function.

LEARNING OBJECTIVES

At the end of the chapter the reader will be able to:

❏ discuss the principles of monitoring *pituitary gland function*;
❏ outline the principles of monitoring the *endocrine function of the pancreas*;
❏ discuss the principles of monitoring *adrenal gland function*;
❏ outline the principles of monitoring *thyroid gland function*;
❏ discuss the principles of monitoring *parathyroid gland function*.

PRINCIPLES OF MONITORING PITUITARY GLAND FUNCTION

One of the functions of the pituitary gland is to secrete the antidiuretic hormone (ADH). ADH acts on the renal tubules resulting in reabsorption of water. Any damage to the posterior pituitary gland or adjacent hypothalamus, for instance following neurosurgery, head injury, malignancy or drug therapy, e.g. amiodarone, can lead to insufficient or lack of ADH secretion (Adam & Osborne 1999) which can lead to diabetes insipidus.

Diabetes insipidus

Diabetes insipidus is a syndrome that has excessive thirst, polydipsia and polyuria as its hallmarks (Vedig 1997a). Water loss in extreme cases can be around 20 litres per day. If untreated diabetes insipidus can result in severe electrolyte imbalance, i.e. severe hypernatraemia and hyperosmolar states.

Monitoring priorities

Management problems on an ICU associated with diabetes insipidus are usually hypovolaemia and polyuria (Vedig 1997a). In respect of hypovolaemia close monitoring of cardiovascular parameters is essential including pulse, blood pressure and central venous pressure monitoring. Maintenance of strict fluid balance and daily weight is also important.

Because patients with diabetes insipidus have an increased serum osmolarity and reduced urine osmolarity, biochemical investigations of both blood and urine are vital in the accurate monitoring of this syndrome.

Specific gravity, a crude measurement, is often ignored on routine ward testing but is invaluable in this case: SG <1.010 is indicative of diabetes insipidus. Urine osmolarity is obtained either as a spot specimen or from a 24h collection. Normal values are 300–1300 mosm/kg.

Plasma osmolarity is calculated from the equation of serum sodium, potassium, glucose and urea (normal value is 275–295 mosm/kg). Regular biochemical assessment of urea and electrolytes is essential to monitor the progression of this syndrome.

PRINCIPLES OF MONITORING THE ENDOCRINE FUNCTION OF THE PANCREAS

The pancreas secretes two hormones, *insulin* and *glucagon*. Functions of insulin include lowering blood glucose levels by promoting transport of glucose into the cells, promoting glycogen storage in muscle and hepatic cells and inhibiting fat metabolism (Adam & Osborne 1999). Glucagon increases blood glucose levels.

Disturbances in pancreatic function that affect insulin production will lead to hyperglycaemia and glycosuria. If left untreated diabetic ketoacidosis will develop.

The normal fasting blood glucose level is 3.9–6.2 mmol/l (Oh 1997). When monitoring a critically ill patient it is important to undertake regular bedside blood glucose measurements, together with urinalysis. These are particularly important if the patient is hypoglycaemic or hyperglycaemic, a known diabetic, receiving insulin or receiving nutritional support.

Monitoring the patient's blood sugar can in the short term prevent hypoglycaemia and ketoacidosis and in the long term prevent disorders that affect the vascular and neural pathways (Mallett & Dougherty 2000).

Blood glucose measurements are more accurate than urinalysis because the results relate to the time of testing (Cowan 1997). The principles of urinalysis have been discussed in Chapter 5. The procedure for bedside blood glucose measurements will now be described.

Procedure for bedside blood glucose measurements

The following is adapted from the Walsall NHS Trust's procedure for 'Blood glucose estimation using the Advantage 11 machine and test strips'.

The procedure for use of the Advantage 11 meter (Fig. 8.1) is as follows.

(1) Wash and dry the patient's hands using soap and water. Avoid using an alcohol swab. It may contaminate the skin and lead to an inaccurate result (Burden 2001).

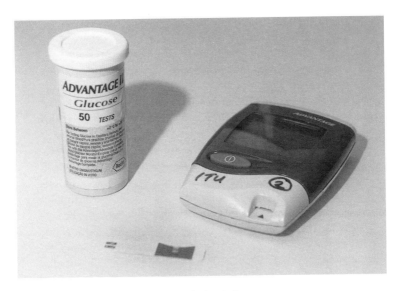

Fig. 8.1 Bedside blood glucose monitoring device

(2) Having ensured the Advantage 11 test strips are in date, remove one from the container and insert it (yellow window facing up) into the test strip slot. The meter should turn on automatically. Replace the container top.

(3) Check that the code number on the meter corresponds to the one on the test strip container. This will help ensure accuracy of the result.

(4) Once the blood drop symbol flashes on the meter, prick the side of the patient's finger with a blood lancet (needles should not be used because they are designed to cut through the skin with minimal trauma resulting in insufficient blood for the test (Burden 2001)). The side of the finger is used because it is less painful for the patient and easier to obtain a hanging droplet of blood (Mallett & Dougherty 2000). As multiple 'stabbing' in the same place

can increase the risk of infection, harden the skin and be painful for the patient the site used should be rotated (Mallett & Dougherty 2000).

(5) After waiting a few seconds to allow the capillaries to relax, squeeze the patient's finger to obtain a small drop of blood, bringing it together with the test strip. The blood will be drawn automatically onto the test strip.

(6) Apply a cotton wool pad or tissue to the patient's finger.

(7) The test result will be displayed in mmol/l after 40s. The presence of a yellow colour in the yellow window following the application of the drop of blood indicates that the test result may be erroneous. Discard the test strip and repeat the procedure.

(8) Document the measurement (Fig. 8.2).

The Advantage 11 test strips should be kept in the original container, stored at room temperature (<32°C) and not refrigerated. Tests should be performed at temperatures between 14 and 40°C.

Best practice – blood glucose measurements

Use soap and water, not alcohol swab, to clean site

Ensure test strip is in date, calibrated with the machine and stored following manufacturer's recommendations

Do not use a needle to draw blood

Use side of patient's finger to draw blood

Rotate finger used to avoid multiple stabbing on the same site

Allow blood to be drawn onto test strip

Ensure sufficient blood has been obtained

Be aware of factors that can affect the result

Ensure quality control procedures are carried out following local protocols

---

WALSALL HOSPITALS NATIONAL HEATH SERVICE TRUST

BLOOD GLUCOSE MONITORING CHART

Patients Name ....

Hospital No. .... Ward ....

DATE & TIME												
28												
24												
22												
20												
18												
16												
15												
14												
13												
12												
11												
10												
09												
08												
07												
06		This area shaded in light blue to indicate near normal range										
05												
04												
03												
02												
01												
Insulin Given												

(left vertical axis label: BLOOD GLUCOSE MMOLS/L)

Fig. 8.2 Blood glucose monitoring chart (Walsall Hospitals NHS Trust)

Blood glucose measurements may be affected by:

- *hyperosmolar hyperglycaemia*: a false low reading may be obtained (Batki *et al.* 1999);
- *hyperlipaemia* (abnormal fat concentrations): e.g. cholesterol > 56.5 mmol/l;
- *high levels of bilirubin* (>0.43 mmol/l: e.g. in jaundice);
- *ascorbic acid (vitamin C) infusion*;
- *peritoneal dialysis*;
- *haemocrit values*: if high (>55%) the blood glucose measurement may be up to 15% too low; if low (<35%) the blood glucose level may be up to 10% too high.
  Medical Devices Agency 1996

To ensure accuracy, quality control procedures using Advantage 11 glucose control solutions should be undertaken following manufacturer's recommendations. The Medical Devices Agency advise that independent quality control procedures should be regularly carried out on all extra-laboratory measurement devices (Medical Devices Agency 1996).

Newer devices are currently being developed to enable non-invasive methods of monitoring blood glucose (Burden 2001). Glucose sensors may give 24 h blood glucose patterns, e.g. to detect unrecognised hypoglycaemia (American Diabetes Association 2001).

Hyperglycaemia and diabetic ketoacidosis

There are many causes of hyperglycaemia including diabetes mellitus, acute pancreatitis, parenteral nutrition and sepsis (Young & Oh 1997).

Diabetic ketoacidosis results from lack of insulin (Watkins 1998). It is a serious life-threatening metabolic complication of diabetes mellitus consisting of three concurrent abnormalities: hyperglycaemia, hyperketonemia and metabolic acidosis (Miller 1999).

A history of infection, illness, inadequate or omitted insulin therapy is common (Kitabchi *et al.* 1983). The characteristics of diabetic ketoacidosis include hyperglycaemia, metabolic acidosis, dehydration, polyuria, glycosuria, ketonuria, weight loss, tachycardia and tachypnoea (Dunning 1994). Monitoring priorities include the following.

- *Airway patency*: (if the patient is semi conscious or in a coma).
- *Arterial blood gas analysis*: patient will be acidotic, breathing may be compromised.
- *Pulse oximetry*: breathing may be compromised.
- *Pulse, blood pressure and central venous pressure measurements*: hypovolaemia.
- *ECG monitoring:* cardiac arrhythmias.
- *Blood glucose measurements*: monitor hyperglycaemia and the effect of prescribed insulin.
- *Urinalysis*: monitor glycosuria and ketonuria.
- *Strict fluid balance*: polyuria and signs of dehydration may be present on physical examination including dry mucous membranes, dry furry tongue, poor skin turgor and soft sunken eyes (Miller 1999). Fluid replacement should be closely monitored.
- *Blood cultures*: to detect sepsis.
- *Serum potassium measurements*: hypokalaemia or hyperkalaemia (Miller 1999).

Hypoglycaemia
Hypoglycaemia, which can be defined as a circulating blood glucose level of <2.0mmol/l (Hinds & Watson 1996), usually occurs in diabetics. Causes include too much insulin or inadequate nutritional intake. It can also complicate hepatic failure, renal failure and adrenocortical insufficiency (Rossini & Mordes 1991, Vedig 1997b). Regular blood glucose measurements are required.

PRINCIPLES OF MONITORING ADRENAL GLAND FUNCTION
The adrenal glands comprise the medulla and cortex. The adrenal medulla secretes the hormones adrenaline and

noradrenaline (catecholamines) in response to sympathetic stimulation. The adrenal cortex secretes three categories of hormones, all of which are steroids.

Phaeochromocytoma

Phaeochromocytoma (tumour of the adrenal medulla) can lead to the secretion of high levels of catecholamines, usually intermittently. Common symptoms include severe hypertension, headache, tachycardia, hyperglycaemia, bowel disturbances and blurred vision (Adam & Osborne 1999). Hypertension is paroxysmal initially, but later becomes sustained (Karet & Brown 1994). Monitoring priorities include:

- *arterial pressure monitoring*: hypertension;
- *ECG monitoring*: cardiac arrhythmias;
- *blood glucose measurements*: to monitor hyperglycaemia and evaluate treatment.

Addisonian crisis

Addisonian crisis results from acute adrenocortisol insufficiency. The clinical features, which relate mainly from the deficiency of aldosterone, include thirst, polyuria, dehydration, cardiac arrhythmias, electrolyte imbalance and hypotension (Adam & Osborne 1999). Monitoring priorities include:

- *arterial blood gas analysis*: metabolic and respiratory acidosis may occur;
- *ECG monitoring*: cardiac arrhythmias;
- *arterial pressure monitoring*: hypotension;
- *central venous pressure monitoring*: hypotension;
- *strict fluid balance*: polyuria;
- *blood glucose measurements*: hypoglycaemia.

PRINCIPLES OF MONITORING THYROID GLAND FUNCTION

The thyroid gland secretes three hormones: *thyroxine* (T3), *triiodothyronine* (T4) and *calcitonin*. T3 and T4 are responsible for the metabolic rate of all bodily tissues. Calcitonin reduces serum calcium levels. Thyroid crisis and myxoedema coma result from over- and undersecretion of the thyroid gland, respectively. If untreated they have a high mortality rate (Vedig 1997c).

Thyroid crisis

Hyperthyroidism (also known as thyrotoxicosis) results from oversecretion of T3 and T4 hormones leading to hyper-metabolism. Thyroid crisis (thyroid storm) is life threatening and is the clinical extreme of hyperthyroidism.

Thyroid crisis is characterised by tachyarrhythmias, hyper-pyrexia, neurological and gastrointestinal disturbances. If the patient has underlying cardiac disease or has a compromised cardiovascular system, the risk of serious complications increases. Thyroid crisis carries a relatively high mortality rate, so careful and accurate monitoring is therefore essential. Monitoring priorities include:

- respiratory rate, pulse oximetry and arterial blood gas analysis: patient may develop pulmonary oedema;
- ECG monitoring: cardiac arrhythmias;
- arterial blood pressure monitoring: hypotension may develop;
- central venous pressure monitoring: patient can develop heart failure, there may also be considerable fluid loss;
- strict fluid balance: considerable fluid loss (excessive sweating);
- blood glucose measurements: hypoglycaemia;
- core temperature measurements: patient may develop extreme pyrexia (>40°C) (Adam & Osborne 1999);
- neurological monitoring: extreme agitation and coma may develop.

Myxoedema coma

Myxoedema coma results from decreased T4 production and occurs most commonly in the elderly female population. There is usually a long history of hypothyroidism (Vedig 1997c). Effects include unconsciousness, hypothermia, hypoventilation, hypotension and hypoglycaemia. Monitoring priorities include:

- *airway*: unconscious patient;
- *respiratory rate, pulse oximetry and arterial blood gas analysis*: hypoventilation;
- *ECG monitoring*: bradycardia;
- *arterial blood pressure monitoring*: hypotension;
- *central venous pressure monitoring*: patient may develop heart failure, also there may be considerable fluid gain;
- *strict fluid balance*: there may be considerable fluid gain;
- *blood glucose measurements*: hypoglycaemia;
- *core temperature measurements*: hypothermia;
- *neurological monitoring*: coma.

PRINCIPLES OF MONITORING PARATHYROID GLAND FUNCTION

The parathyroid glands secrete the parathyroid hormone which raises serum calcium levels. Calcium is essential for a variety of bodily functions including muscle contraction, blood clotting and maintenance of cell membrane integrity. Abnormalities in parathyroid function (hyperparathyroidism and hypoparathyroidism) can lead to calcium disorders which can be life threatening.

Hypercalcaemia

Symptomatic hypercalcaemia requires urgent treatment and if it is severe the patient should be admitted to the ICU (Adam & Osborne 1999). Monitoring priorities include:

- *ECG monitoring*: cardiac arrhythmias;
- *arterial blood pressure monitoring*: hypertension;
- *central venous pressure monitoring*: hypovolaemia;
- *strict fluid balance*: dehydration, polyuria and hypovolaemia.

Hypocalcaemia

Acute hypocalcaemia complicated by tetany, convulsions and cardiovascular problems requires urgent treatment (Scheinkestel & Oh 1997). Monitoring priorities include:

- *airway patency*;
- *respirations, pulse oximetry and arterial blood gas analysis*: respiratory compromise;
- *ECG monitoring*: cardiac arrhythmias;
- *arterial blood pressure*: hypotension;
- *central venous pressure monitoring*: hypotension;
- *neurological monitoring*: convulsions and altered conscious level.

Scenario

Mr Jones, a 28-year-old man, was admitted to the medical HDU with a history of weight loss, general malaise, polyuria, polydipsia, lethargy and deep sighing Kussmaul respirations. He was a known diabetic but had omitted his insulin injections over the preceding few days and was also complaining of diarrhoea and vomiting. A provisional diagnosis of diabetic ketoacidosis was made. What are the monitoring priorities?

BP 90/60, pulse 125, resps 35, temp 38.5°C, SpO$_2$ 95%, blood glucose is 40 mmol. The patient's vital signs were consistent with acute circulatory failure secondary to dehydration caused by excessive fluid loss. The pyrexia may be associated with the diarrhoea and vomiting. Blood glucose measurements and urinalysis were undertaken. The presence of hyperglycaemia, glycosuria, ketonuria and ketonaemia helped to confirm the diagnosis of diabetic ketoacidosis.

Arterial blood gas results are as follows:

pH 7.1

PCO$_2$ 2.9

PO$_2$ 11.8

HCO$_3$ 12

BE −13

SaO$_2$ 97%

What do the arterial blood gases show?

The patient has metabolic acidosis with respiratory compensation. He is hyperventilating in order to excrete more CO$_2$, therefore reducing the level of free hydrogen ions available.

Strict fluid balance monitoring was started. Fluid replacement was started together with an insulin infusion to treat the hyperglycaemia. ECG monitoring was essential as hypokalaemia (K = 2.8 mmol/l) was present. Potassium IV replacement therapy was also commenced. Ongoing monitoring priorities include vital signs, arterial blood gases, ECG monitoring, blood glucose measurements, urinalysis, fluid balance and any vomiting/bowel action. In addition it is important to monitor the patient's conscious level as unconsciousness may ensue.

CONCLUSION

Monitoring endocrine function is an important aspect of caring for the critically ill patient. Brief details on normal physiology, in relation to each endocrine gland function, have been provided. The priorities of monitoring endocrine function have been highlighted.

REFERENCES

Adam, S. & Osborne, S. (1999) *Critical Care Nursing: Science and Practice*. Oxford Medical Publications, Oxford.

American Diabetes Association (2001) Clinical practice recommendations. *Diabetes Care* **24**, (Supplement) S80–S82.

Batki, A., Holder, R., Thomason, H. *et al.* (1999) Selecting blood glucose monitoring systems. *Professional Nurse* **14** (10), 715–723.

Burden, M. (2001) Diabetes: blood glucose monitoring. *Nursing Times* **97** (8), 37–39.

Cowan, T. (1997) Blood glucose monitoring devices. *Professional Nurse* **12** (8), 593–597.

Dunning, T. (1994) *Care of People with Diabetes*. Blackwell Science, Oxford.

Hinds, C.J. & Watson, D. (1996) *Intensive Care: A Concise Textbook*, 2nd edn. W.B. Saunders, London.

Karet, F. & Brown, M. (1994) Phaeochromocytoma: diagnosis and management. *Postgraduate Medical Journal* **70**, 326–328.

Kitabchi, A., Fisher, J., Matteri, R. & Murphy, M. (1983) The use of continuous insulin delivery systems in the treatment of diabetes mellitus. *Advances in International Medicine* **28**, 449–490.

Mallett, J. & Dougherty, L. (2000) eds *The Royal Marsden Hospital Manual of Clinical Nursing Procedures*. Blackwell Science, Oxford.

Medical Devices Agency Adverse Incident Centre (1996) Safety Notice 9616: Extra-laboratory use of blood glucose meters and test strips: contra-indications, training and advice to users. Medical Devices Agency, London.

Miller, J. (1999) Management of diabetic ketoacidosis. *Journal of Emergency Nursing* **25** (6), 514–519.

Oh, T. (1997) ed. *Intensive Care Manual*, 4th edn. Butterworth Heinemann, Oxford.

Rossini, A. & Mordes, J. (1991) *The diabetic comas*. In: J. Rippe, R. Irwin., J. Albert & M. Fink eds, *Intensive Care Medicine*. Little Brown, Boston.

Scheinkestel, C. & Oh, T. (1997) Acute calcium disorders. In: T. Oh, ed. *Intensive Care Manual*, 4th edn. Butterworth Heinemann, Oxford.

Vedig, A. (1997a) Diabetes insipidus. In: T. Oh, ed. *Intensive Care Manual*, 4th edn. Butterworth Heinemann, Oxford.

Vedig, A. (1997b) Adrenocortical insufficiency. In: T. Oh, ed. *Intensive Care Manual*, 4th edn. Butterworth Heinemann, Oxford.

Vedig, A. (1997c) Thyroid emergencies. In: T. Oh, ed. *Intensive Care Manual*, 4th edn. Butterworth Heinemann, Oxford.

Watkins, P. (1998) *ABC of Diabetes*, 4th edn. BMJ Publishing Group, London.

Young, K. & Oh, T. (1997) Diabetic emergencies In: T. Oh, ed. *Intensive Care Manual*, 4th edn. Butterworth Heinemann, Oxford.

Monitoring
Nutritional Status

9

INTRODUCTION

A survey carried out by McWhirter and Pennington (1994) found that 40% of patients were malnourished during their stay in hospital. Both medical and nursing staff often fail to assess and monitor nutritional status (Lennard-Jones *et al.* 1995), particularly in ICU patients (Adam, 1994 and Briggs 1996). Malnutrition is prevalent in many ventilated patients and its incidence on the ICU could be as high as 50% (McCain 1993).

Recent studies, however, have demonstrated that malnourished patients have poorer outcomes following medical treatment or surgery (Kennedy 1997 and Say 1997), particularly those with a weight loss greater than 10%. The commencement of early nutritional support together with on-going monitoring of nutritional status is therefore now considered a high priority.

The aim of this chapter is to understand the principles of monitoring nutritional status.

LEARNING OBJECTIVES

At the end of the chapter the reader will be able to:

❏ discuss the *importance* of assessing nutritional status;
❏ outline *how to assess* nutritional status;
❏ list the factors that can *affect* nutritional status;
❏ discuss the principles of monitoring *enteral feeding*; and
❏ discuss the principles of monitoring *parenteral nutrition*.

IMPORTANCE OF ASSESSING NUTRITIONAL STATUS

All critically ill patients have either a serious illness, have suffered major trauma and/or have had major surgery; the stress response to trauma and/or injury results in a hypermetabolic state and increased nutritional demands (Verity 1996).

Severe protein-calorie malnutrition is the main problem in many ICU patients because of the high catabolic rate associated with acute critical illness and the common presence of previous chronic wasting conditions (Webb *et al.* 1999).

The effects of absent nutritional intake in critically ill patients include mucosal atrophy, loss of body tissue, skeletal muscle atrophy and weakness, immunosuppresion and delayed wound healing (Verity 1996); these effects may occur within days (Farquhar 1993). In particular it is now recognised that maintaining gut integrity is important to help prevent sepsis and to support the immune defence system (Albarran & Price 1998).

ASSESSMENT OF THE PATIENT'S NUTRITIONAL STATUS

Bedside nutritional assessment should identify patients already suffering from malnutrition and those at risk of malnutrition; early referral for nutritional support together with ongoing monitoring is essential.

Objectives of assessment

The objectives of this assessment are to:

- determine the existing *nutritional status* of the patient;
- identify if the patient is *malnourished*;
- provide a baseline for *monitoring* nutritional status;
- ascertain the patient's *nutritional requirements*.

Assessment

There is no gold standard for determining the nutritional status of patients (Arrowsmith 1999). However as any one single method can have shortcomings, it it recommended to use two or three methods in parallel to overcome this problem (McLaren & Green 1998 and Quirk 2000). The different methods of nutritional assessment in patients requiring intensive care will now be discussed.

A 24h recall of dietary intake, food diaries and taking a dietary history are all frequently used in clinical practice (Arrowsmith 1999). A diet history can provide information on food frequency, food preferences, food allergies, portion sizes and changes in food intake.

A clinical examination can help to determine whether nutrition is inadequate (Dobb 1997) and recommended simple measurements include:

- height;
- weight;
- mid-upper-arm circumferences (low = overall weight loss);
- triceps skinfold thickness (low = significant depletion of fat stores);
- mid-arm muscle circumference (= protein depletion).

Woodrow 2000

Regular measurements of skinfold thickness can provide an indication of oedema or dehydration and whether fat is being used as an energy source. However in the critically ill patient this measurement may be unreliable (Taylor & Goodinson-McLaren 1992).

The patient's body mass index (BMI) can be used to calculate the nutritional status of the patient (Albarran & Price 1998). This is determined by the patient's weight and height. Nomograms are available that can aid calculation. Unfortunately regular BMI estimations are difficult in critically ill patients (Endacott 1993).

The measurement of serum albumin levels is not a good indicator of nutritional status (Horwood 1990), because a fall is more likely to result from albumin's metabolism, reflecting

Table 9.1 The Harris–Benedict equation for calculating basal metabolic rate (taken from Quirk 2000)

Men	Energy expenditure = $66.5 + (13.7 \times$ weight) $+ 5 \times$ (height) $- 6.78 \times$ (age in years)
Women	Energy expenditure = $66.5 + (9.56 \times$ weight in kg) $+ 1.85 \times$ (height in cm) $- 4.68 \times$ (age in years)
Injury factors	Minor operation $\times 1.2$ Trauma $\times 1.3$ Sepsis $\times 1.6$ Severe burns $\times 2.1$

the severity and duration of stress, rather than nutritional status (Quirk 2000).

Muscle atrophy may be masked by gross oedema and deceptive increases in body weight (Say 1997) and can also result from prolonged immobility. Urinalysis (presence of ketones) and blood glucose monitoring are helpful.

Metabolic monitoring using indirect calorimetry may be useful. An open circuit metabolic monitor, attached to the ventilator, can sample inspiratory and expiratory O_2 and CO_2 and can provide a continuous measurement of energy expenditure (Adam 1994). However it is inaccurate if the patient is receiving oxygen concentrations of 60% or more (Albarran & Price 1998).

There are a number of empirical formulas and nomograms that can be used to calculate the basal metabolic rate, the Harris–Benedict (1919) equation (Table 9.1) being the most well-known (Quirk 2000). However in critically ill patients baseline calculation errors can occur because the ideal weight and height is rarely known (Quirk 2000).

FACTORS THAT CAN AFFECT NUTRITIONAL STATUS

Common factors that can affect nutritional status in critically ill patients include:

- inability to take oral diet;
- diarrhoea;
- glucose intolerance;
- renal dysfunction;
- pain;
- nausea/vomiting;
- physical disability;
- restricted fluid intake;
- delayed gastric emptying;
- fasting prior to procedures/investigations.

PRINCIPLES OF MONITORING ENTERAL FEEDING

If the patient is able to take diet and fluids orally, it is important to monitor intake closely to ensure that hydration and nutritional needs are being met. Sip-feed supplements, e.g. Complan, Build Up, may improve clinical outcome (Larsson *et al.* 1990) and food charts are useful as long as they are accurately completed.

If food and sip feeding fails to meet nutritional requirements or if the patient is unable to tolerate oral diet, enteral feeding should be considered. Enteral feeding, defined as the administration of nutrients via the gastrointestinal tract (Bruce & Finley 1997), should always be used whenever possible (Dobb 1992).

Benefits of enteral feeding

Benefits of enteral feeding include:

- improved function of the gut and liver;
- enhanced immune function, reduced infection rates and lower sepsis rates compared to parenteral feeding (Moore *et al.* 1992 and Leary *et al.* 2000);
- possible prevention of bacterial translocation (passage of bacteria or endotoxins across the intestinal epithelium to the portal venous lymphatics, which may lead to sepsis) (Botterill & MacFie 2000);

- improved survival rates in critically ill patients (Methany 1996);
- promotion of wound healing (Heyland 1998).

Methods of enteral feeding

There are several methods of enteral feeding:

- *nasogastric*: tube through the nose into the stomach;
- *nasoenteric*: tube through the nose into the jejunum or duodenum;
- *gastrostomy or jejunostomy*: tube surgically or percutaneously inserted into the stomach or jejunum.

Nasogastric feeding

Nasogastric feeding is often started through a wide-bore (12–14FG) tube. This allows aspiration of gastric contents to confirm tube placement and feed tolerance and facilitates the administration of medications. They are less likely to occlude compared to fine-bore tubes, but their long-term use is not recommended. Following insertion of a wide-bore tube, which should be radio opaque so that the tip can be visualised on a chest X-ray, it is important to ensure correct tube placement by observing the following precautions.

- Auscultating over the stomach following injection of air via the tube: this method may only be 60% reliable (Methany *et al*. 1990).
- Aspirating gastric contents and testing the pH; if the NG tube is in the stomach and in contact with acidic gastric contents the aspirate will turn blue litmus paper red. **NB** the result may be affected if the patient is taking H_2 agonists or if the NG tube is in the duodenum (Adam 1994).

Continuous enteral feeding reduces gastric acidity and increases the risk of pneumonia (Jacobs *et al*. 1990 and Lee *et al*. 1990). Rest periods are therefore recommended, usually of at least four hours (Goldhill 2000) though at present there is no evidence determining the optimum length of time (Woodrow 2000).

Aspiration of gastric contents should be undertaken every 4–6 h to assess gastric residual volume and provide an indication to feed tolerance. This is particularly important in the initial period when enteral feeding is being established (Raper & Maynard 1992). If the patient vomits it is usual practice to continue the feed at 10 ml per hour.

In addition aspiration is usually undertaken one hour following the interruption of feeding, by which time gastric emptying should have occurred (Woodrow 2000). Discarding aspirated volumes may cause an electrolyte imbalance (Methany 1993). It is therefore recommended to return all aspirate of <200 ml via the nasogastric tube (Goldhill 2000). Patients who are ventilated may have normal gastric emptying despite the lack of bowel sounds (Shelly & Church 1987). Opiates and increased intracranial pressure can impair gastric emptying (Norton *et al.* 1988).

Complications associated with wide-bore tubes include the following.

- *Nasal/oesophageal ulceration and airway/gastrointestinal haemorrhage*: more prevalent than with fine-bore tubes (Bettany & Powell-Tuck 1997).
- *Transbronchial insertion*: misplacement rates vary between 0.9% (Methany *et al.* 1990) and 2.4% (Payne-James 1988).
- *Sinusitis.*
- *Regurgitation and aspiration of gastric contents*: particularly in unconscious and ventilated patients. The presence of a nasogastric tube renders the gastro-oesophageal sphincter incompetent allowing reflux of gastric contents; a cuffed endotracheal tube does not guarantee 100% protection from aspiration (Hinds & Watson 1996). The nurse should be alert to the possibility of aspiration and should monitor the patient's respiratory function together with the consistency of suction contents.

- *Tube migration*: the tube should be well secured and marked to facilitate the early detection of migration; it should also be regularly monitored (Methany 1993). The blue litmus test on aspirated gastric contents should be undertaken regularly.
- *Risk of nosocomial pneumonia* as wide bore tubes facilitate the migration of gut commensals into the respiratory tract particularly in the presence of H_2 blockers.
- *Tube blockage*.

Nasoenteric feeding

Nasoenteric feeding requires the use of fine-bore tubes, which are better tolerated by patients, can remain *in situ* for longer periods and cause less mucosal erosion and irritation (Raper & Maynard 1992). The feed is usually continuous and administered at a slower rate because the small intestine is unable to tolerate sudden rate changes or bolus feedings (Grodner *et al.* 1996).

Correct tube placement must be confirmed by radiography (Moxham & Goldstone 1994). Unfortunately fine-bore tubes can collapse following the application of negative pressure by a syringe, thus making them more difficult to aspirate. This may lead to decreased nursing vigilance in assessing gastric contents (Sands 1991).

Complications associated with fine-bore tubes include the following.

- *Misplacement*: 0.3–4.0% of insertions (Dobb 1997).
- *Tube migration* (Biggart *et al.* 1987): coughing and vomiting can dislodge the tube, increasing the risk of aspiration (Kennedy 1997). Check the gastric pH if high reflux is present or if H_2 antagonists are being used.
- *Guide-wire induced trauma*: e.g. oesophageal, gastric and abdominal perforation and a pneumothorax.
- *Tube blockage*.

As the tube is placed past the pylorus (gastric-duodenal sphincter), the risk of regurgitation and aspiration of gastric contents is reduced (Hudak *et al.* 1998).

Complications of enteral feeding

Complications of enteral feeding are more commonly associated with patients requiring intensive care (Dobb 1990). The most significant ones are listed below.

- *Regurgitation and aspiration of gastric contents*: this is more common in the unconscious patient, supine patient (Ibanez *et al.* 1992) and older patient (Mullen *et al.* 1992). The presence of a wide-bore tube renders the gastro-oesophageal sphincter incompetent (Hinds & Watson 1996). Nurses need to observe suction. If possible, the patient's 'head end' should be maintained at 45 degrees.
- *Tube obstruction*: if the feed is stopped, the tube should be flushed with 10–20 ml of sterile water; if the tube is not in use it should be capped off after flushing in order to trap a column of water in the tube (Taylor 1988).
- *Diarrhoea*: associated with hyperosmolar feed and antibiotic usage.
- *Abdominal distension*: if there is poor gastric emptying, rapid infusion of feed. This is also an indication of failure to absorb the feed; careful monitoring is essential in order to prevent perforation of the intestines (Raper & Maynard 1992).
- Hyperglycaemia.
- Mild hepatic dysfunction.

Best practice – nasogastric feeding

Use fine bore tube whenever possible

Always confirm tube position before commencement of feed

Monitor tube position during feeding

Monitor the patient's vital signs, particularly airway

Administer feed following local guidelines ensuring breaks as appropriate

Ensure feed is in date and administered following manufacturer's recommendations

Monitor absorption of feed

Always use clean syringe and receptacle when aspirating

Maintain fluid balance

Monitor bowel function

Monitor patient's blood chemistry

Percutaneous jejunostomy and percutaneous endoscopic gastrostomy (PEG)

PEG is the preferred method for long-term access to the GI tract (Pollard 2000). Complications include leaks, wound infection and peritonitis (Adams *et al.* 1986). The insertion site should be closely monitored, particularly as gastric contents can leak around it leading to excoriation, skin breakdown and possible wound dehiscence (Kennedy 1997). Misplacement of the tube can occur leading to peritonitis.

PRINCIPLES OF MONITORING PARENTERAL NUTRITION

Parenteral nutrition (PN) (Fig. 9.1) is the preferred terminology to total parenteral nutrition (TPN) (Hamilton 2000). PN involves the intravenous infusion of nutrients. It should only be considered when the gastrointestinal tract is not functioning, e.g. in acute pancreatitis, peritonitis, malabsorption syndromes and paralytic ileus. It can be administered either peripherally or centrally, but has not been shown to reduce mortality (Heyland 1998).

Table 9.2 provides a comprehensive guide to the relevant monitoring required when a patient is receiving PN. In particular the nurse should be alert to the possible complications of PN, which can cause death in 0.2% of patients (Wolfe *et al.* 1986).

During PN administration, there is a significant risk of mor-

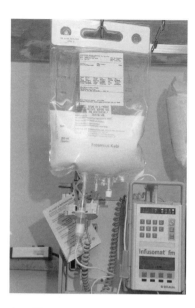

Fig. 9.1 Parenteral nutrition

bidity through catheter-related sepsis and also metabolic and mechanical problems (Heenan 1996). Infection is the biggest problem (Phillips 1997), with infection rates for PN catheters as high as 6%, compared to 1.5% for jejunostomy tubes (Schears & Deutschman 1997). Careful aseptic techniques are paramount (McGee *et al.* 1993); the entire infusion line should be dedicated to PN use, unnecessary manipulation of the line and use of three-way stopcocks is not recommended (Phillips 1997).

Hyperosmolar dehydration syndrome can complicate hyperglycaemia; urine levels of glucose of > 2% and a sudden rise in urine volumes are clinical features of osmotic diuresis (Phillips 1997). In addition, rebound hypoglycaemia can occur if the PN infusions are abruptly stopped. Regular urinalysis and blood glucose monitoring is therefore important.

The function of the gut should be monitored so that

Table 9.2 Parenteral nutrition – relevant monitoring

Regular clinical	Nursing observations
	Temperature
	Blood pressure
	Pulse rate
	Respiratory rate
	Fluid balance
Regular ward testing	Medical assessment
	Urinalysis
	Dextrostix
	Reflectance meter
	Blood glucose
Daily (at least)	Fluid balance review
	Nutrient input review
	Biochemistry
	Serum electrolytes
	Serum urea/creatinine
	Blood glucose
Weekly (at least)	Complete blood count
	Coagulation screen
	Weight
	Liver functions tests
	Serum calcium/magnesium/phosphate
As indicated	Serum lipids
	Urine zinc
	Serum uric acid
	Blood gases
	24-h urinary urea, electrolytes, osmolality
Special circumstances	Nitrogen balance
	Body composition
	Body protein turnover
	Gas exchange measurements
	Trace element balance
	Vitamin assays

Reproduced by permission of Butterworth-Heinemann from Oh 1997

conversion to enteral nutrition can be initiated as soon as possible. PN should be gradually withdrawn in order to avoid complications, e.g. rebound hypoglycaemia (Phillips 1997). If

PN is delivered intermittently the catheter should be flushed with heparinised normal saline in order to minimise the risk of clot formation (Cottee 1995).

Best practice – parenteral feeding

Only use when enteral route is not possible

Do not use feed bag if there are signs of contamination

Administer feed following local protocols

Ensure entire infusion line is dedicated to PN use

Ensure feed and tubing is regularly changed

Monitor patient's blood chemistry

Monitor patient for complications of PN, particularly infection

Regularly flush line when not in use to maintain patency

Monitor gut function so that enteral feeding can be commenced as soon as possible

---

Scenario

Mr Brown was admitted to the ICU with an atypical pneumonia. He was sedated and ventilated with midazolam and morphine. A fine-bore naso gastric tube was inserted and the position verified by the litmus paper test and X-ray. Enteral feeding was then commenced (standard feed) at 30 ml/ h. After four hours 100 ml is aspirated. What would you do?

As the aspirate is < 200 ml, it is replaced because of its constituents:

- *gastric acid* reduces the proliferation of bacteria;
- *gastrin promotes* the growth and repair of the gastric mucosa;
- *intrinsic factor* facilitates the absorption of Vit B12 from the gut.

The enteral feed was increased to 60 ml/ h. After four hours 300 ml was aspirated. What would you do?

200 ml was replaced while 100 ml was discarded and the feed reduced to 30 ml/ h. After four hours 400 ml was aspirated. Again 200 ml was replaced and the rest discarded. The enteral feed was then re-started at 30 ml/ h. Shortly after

recommencement of the feed, the patient vomited. What would you do?

Nil was aspirated and the feed was reduced to 10 ml/h continuously and the prokinetic drug metoclopramide 10 mg I/V prescribed three times daily. The following day the feed was gradually increased following the above process until a desired rate of 90 ml/h was reached. Eight-hourly monitoring of aspirate, urea and electrolytes, fluid balance and bowel movements ensured a successful enteral feeding regime.

CONCLUSION

Nutritional status should be assessed and monitored in all critically ill patients. The method of nutritional support should also be closely monitored, in particular the patient's tolerance of it. The nurse should also be alert to possible complications.

REFERENCES

Adam, S. (1994) Aspects of current research in enteral nutrition in the critically ill. *Care of the Critically Ill* **10** (6), 246–251.

Adams, M., Seabrook, G., Quebbeman, E. & Condon, R. (1986) Jejunostomy: a rarely indicated procedure *Annals of Surgery* **121**, 236–238.

Albarran, J. & Price, T. (1998) *Managing the Nursing Priorities in Intensive Care*. Quay Books/Mark Allen Publishing, Dinton.

Allison, S. (1984) Nutritional problems in intensive care. *Hospital Update* **10** (12), 1001–1012.

Arrowsmith, H. (1999) A critical evaluation of the use of nutritional screening tools by nurses. *British Journal of Nursing* **8** (22), 1483–1490.

Bettany, G. & Powell-Tuck, J. (1997) Nutritional support in surgery. *Surgery* **15** (10), 233–237.

Biggart, M., McQuillan, P., Choudhry, A. & Nickalls, R. (1987) Dangers of placement of narrow-bore nasogastric feeding tubes. *Annals of the Royal College of Surgeons of England* **69**, 119–121.

Botterill, I. & MacFie, J. (2000) Bacterial translocation in the critically ill: a review of the evidence. *Care of the Critically Ill* **16** (1), 6–11.

Briggs, D. (1996) Nasogastric feeding in intensive care units: a study. *Nursing Standard* **49** (10), 42–45.

Bruce, L. & Finley, T.M.D. (1997) *Nursing in Gastroenterology*. Churchill Livingstone, London.

Cottee, S. (1995) Heparin lock practice in total parenteral nutrition. *Professional Nurse* **11** (1), 25–29.

Dobb, G. (1990) Enteral nutrition *Clinical Anaesthesiology* **4**, 531–557.

Dobb, G. (1992) Enteral nutrition for the critically ill. In: J. Vincent, ed. *Yearbook of Intensive Care and Emergency Medicine*. Springer-Verlag, Berlin.

Dobb, G. (1997) Enteral nutrition. In: T. Oh, ed. *Intensive Care Manual*, 4th edn. Butterworth Heinemann, Oxford.

Endacott, R. (1993) Nutritional support for critically ill patients. *Nursing Standard* **7**(52), 25–28.

Farquhar, I. (1993) Parenteral nutrition in the critically ill. *Current Anaesthesia and Critical Care* **4**, 95–102.

Goldhill, D. (2000) Feeding critically ill patients. *Care of the Critically Ill* **16** (1), 20–21.

Grodner, M., Long Anderson, S., de Young, S. *et al.* (1996) *Foundations and Clinical Applications of. Nutrition: A Nursing Approach.* Mosby Yearbook, St Louis MO.

Hamilton, H. (2000) *Total Parenteral Nutrition*. Churchill Livingstone, London.

Harris, J. & Benedict, F. (1919) *A Biometric Study of Basal Metabolism in Man.* Carnegie Institute, Washington DC.

Heenan, A. (1996) Fluids used in total parenteral nutrition. *Professional Nurse* **7**, 467–470.

Heyland, D. (1998) Nutritional support in the critically ill patient. *Critical Care Clinics* **14** (3), 423–440.

Hinds, C.J. & Watson, D. (1996) *Intensive Care: A Concise Textbook*, 2nd edn. W.B. Saunders, London.

Horwood, A. (1990) Malnourishment in intensive care units as high as 50%: are nurses doing enough to change this? *Intensive Care Nursing* **8** (3), 185–188.

Hudak, C.M., Gallo, B.M. & Morton, P.G. (1998) *Critical Care Nursing a holistic approach*, 7th edn. Lippincott, New York.

Ibanez, J., Penafiel, A., Raurich, J. *et al.* (1992) Gastroesophageal reflux (GER) in intubated patients receiving enteral nutrition: effect of supine and semirecumbent positions. *Journal of Parenteral and Enteral Nutrition* **16**, 419–422.

Jacobs, S., Chang, R., Lee, B. *et al.* (1990) Continuous enteral feeding: a major cause of pneumonia among ventilated patients. *Journal of Parenteral and Enteral Nutrition* **14**, 353–356.

Kennedy, J. (1997) Enteral feeding for the critically ill patient. *Nursing Standard* **11** (33), 39–43.

Larca, L. & Greenbaum, D. (1982) Effectiveness of intensive nutritional regimes in patients who fail to wean from mechanical ventilation. *Critical Care Medicine* **10**, 297–300.

Larsson, J., Knossan, M., Er, A. *et al.* (1990) Effect of dietary supplement on nutritional status and clinical outcome in 501 geriatric patients: a randomised study. *Clinical Nutrition* **9** (4), 179–184.

Leary, T., Fellows, I. & Fletcher, S. (2000) Enteral nutrition. *Care of the Critically Ill* **16** (1), 22–27.

Lee, B., Chang, R. & Jacobs, S. (1990) Intermittent nasogastric feeding: a simple and effective method to reduce pneumonia among ventilated ICU patients. *Clinical Intensive Care* **1** (3), 100–102.

Lennard-Jones, J., Arrowsmith, H., Davison, C. *et al.* (1995) Screening by nurses and junior doctors to detect malnutrition when patients are first assessed in hospital. *Clinical Nutrition* **14**, 336–340.

Levinson, M. & Bryce, A. (1993) Enteral feeding, gastric colonisation and diarrhoea in critically ill patients: is there a relationship? *Anaesthesia and Intensive Care* **21** (1), 85–88.

Mallett, J. & Dougherty, L. (2000) eds *The Royal Marsden Hospital Manual of Clinical Nursing Procedures*. Blackwell Science, Oxford.

McCain, R. (1993) A sensible approach to the nutritional support of mechanically ventilated critically ill patients. *Intensive Care Medecine* **19**, 129–139.

McClave, S., Snider, H., Lowen, C. *et al.* (1992) Use of residual volume as a marker for enteral feeding intolerance: prospective blinded comparison with physical examination and radiographic findings. *Journal of Parenteral and Enteral Nutrition* **16**, 419–422.

McGee, W., Ackerman, B., Rouben, L. *et al.* (1993) Accurate placement of central venous catheters: a prospective, randomised, multi-center trial. *Critical Care Medicine* **21**, 1118–1123.

McLaren, S. & Green, S. (1998) Nutritional screening and assessment. *Professional Nurse* **13** (6), Study Supplement, S9–S14.

McWhirter, J. & Pennington, C. (1994) Incidence and recognition of malnutrition in hospital. *British Medical Journal* **308**, 945–948.

Methany, N. (1993) Minimising respiratory complications of nasogastric tube feedings: state of the science. *Heart and Lung* **22** (3), 213–222.

Methany, N. (1996) *Fluid and Electrolyte Balance: Nursing Considerations*, 3rd edn. Lippincott, Philadelphia.

Methany, N., Dettenmeier, P., Hampton, K. *et al.* (1990) Detection of inadvertent respiratory placement of small-bore feeding tubes: a report of 10 cases. *Heart and Lung* **19**, 631–638.

Moore, F., Feliciano, D., Andrassy, R. *et al.* (1992) Early enteral feeding, compared with parenteral, reduces postoperative septic complications. *Annals of Surgery* **216** (2), 172–183.

Moxham, J. & Goldstone, J. (1994) *Assisted Ventilation* 3rd edn. BMJ Publishing, London.

Mullen, H., Roubenoff, R.A. & Roubenoff, A. (1992) Risk of pulmonary aspiration among patients receiving enteral nutritional support. *Journal of Parenteral and Enteral Nutrition* **16**, 160–164.

Norton, J., Ott, L., McClain, C. *et al.* (1988) Intolerance to enteral feeding in the brain injured patient. *Journal of Neurosurgery* **68**, 62–66.

Oh, T. (ed.) (1997) *Intensive Care Manual*, 4th edn. Butterworth-Heinemann, Oxford.

Payne-James, J. (1988) Enteral nutrition: clinical applications. *Intensive Therapy and Clinical Monitoring* **7**, 239–246.

Phillips, G. (1997) Parenteral nutrition. In: T. Oh ed., *Intensive Care Manual* 4th edn. Butterworth-Heinemann, Oxford.

Pollard, C. (2000) A PEG service with nurses at its heart. *Nursing Times* **96** (39), 39–40.

Quirk, J. (2000) Malnutrition in critically ill patients in intensive care units. *British Journal of Nursing* **9** (9), 537–541.

Raper, S. & Maynard, N. (1992) Feeding the critically ill patient. *British Journal of Nursing* **1** (6), 273–280.

Sands, J. (1991) Incidence of pulmonary aspiration in intubated patients receiving enteral nutrition through wide- and narrow-bore nasogastric feeding tubes. *Heart Lung* **20**, 75–80.

Say, J. (1997) Nutritional assessment in clinical practice: a review. *Nursing in Critical Care* **2** (1) 29–33.

Schears, G. & Deutschman, C. (1997) Common nutritional issues in paediatric and adult critical care medicine. *Critical Care Clinics* **13** (3), 669–690.

Shelly, M. & Church, J. (1987) Bowel sounds during intermittent positive pressure ventilation. *Anaesthesia* **42**, 207–209.

Solomon, S. & Kirby, D. (1990) The refeeding syndrome: a review. *Journal of Parenteral and Enteral Nutrition* **14**, 90–97.

Taylor, S. (1988) A guide to nasogastric feeding equipment. *Professional Nurse* **4**, 91–94.

Taylor, S. & Goodinson-McLaren, S. (1992) *Nutritional Support: A Team Approach.* Wolfe Publishing, London.

Verity, S. (1996) Nutrition and its importance to intensive care patients. *Intensive and Critical Care Nursing* **12**, 71–78.

Webb, A., Shapiro, M., Singer, M. & Surter, P. (1999) *The Oxford Textbook of Critical Care.* Oxford Medical, Oxford.

Wolfe, B., Ryder, M., Nishikawa, R. *et al.* (1986) Complications of parenteral nutrition. *American Journal of Surgery* **152**, 93–99.

Woodrow, P. (2000) *Intensive Care Nursing: A Framework for Practice.* Routledge, London.

Monitoring Temperature

INTRODUCTION

The body can only function effectively within a narrow temperature range (Woodrow 2000). Any significant changes in temperature, either increases or decreases, can lead to life-threatening complications. As a critically ill patient can experience wide fluctuations in temperature, close temperature monitoring is paramount.

Monitoring temperature is particularly important if the patient has a condition that affects basal metabolic rate, e.g. thyrotoxicosis, is susceptible to infection, e.g. neutropenic, already has a local or systemic infection, is receiving a blood transfusion or is in the postoperative phase.

The aim of this chapter is to understand the principles of monitoring temperature.

LEARNING OBJECTIVES

At the end of this chapter the reader will be able to

❏ discuss the factors *influencing* body temperature;
❏ discuss the methods of *measuring* temperature;
❏ discuss the physiological effects of *hypothermia*;
❏ outline the *monitoring priorities* of a patent with *hypothermia*;
❏ discuss the *physiological effects* of hyperthermia;
❏ outline the *monitoring priorities* of a patient with *hyperthermia*.

FACTORS INFLUENCING BODY TEMPERATURE

The normal body temperature is usually between 36 and 37.5°C , regardless of the environmental temperature (Marinin

& Wheeler 1997). Temperature is regulated by the thermoregulatory centre in the hypothalamus through various physiological mechanisms, e.g. sweating, dilation/constriction of peripheral blood vessels and shivering.

The body's core temperature is usually the highest, while the skin's is the coolest. Core temperature represents the balance between the heat generated by body tissues during metabolic activity, especially of the liver and muscles, and heat lost during various *mechanisms* (Mallett & Dougherty 2000).

There are four mechanisms of heat loss (Tappen & Andre 1996):

- *radiation*: flow of heat from a higher temperature (the body) to a lower temperature (environment surrounding the body);
- *convection*: heat transfer by flow or movement of air;
- *conduction*: heat transfer due to direct contact with cooler surfaces;
- *evaporation*: perspiration, respiration and breaks in skin integrity.

There are a number of factors that can cause a fluctuation in temperature including:

- The body's *circadian rhythms*: temperature is higher in the evening than the morning (Brown 1990), the difference can be as much as 1.5°C (Minor & Waterhouse 1981). If temperature is being recorded every 4–6h, the optimum time for detecting a pyrexia is probably between 7pm and 8pm (Angerami 1980).
- *Ovulation*.
- *Exercise* and *eating* can cause a rise in temperature (Marieb 1998).
- *Old age*: there is an increased sensitivity to the cold and there is generally a lower body temperature.
- *Illness*.

METHODS OF MEASURING TEMPERATURE

The traditional method of using oral/rectal mercury thermometers is now seldom used (Kelly *et al*. 2001). Mercury is covered by the Control of Substances Hazardous to Health Regulations (COSHH) 1999 and its vapour is neurotoxic (Woodrow 2000). In addition, although rectal temperature is closest to core temperature (Schmitz *et al*. 1994), it is unreliable in the critically ill patient because hypotension and gut ischaemia reduce the blood supply to the rectum (Holtzclaw 1992) and the measurement is influenced by the contents in the rectum.

However, there are several reliable methods of measuring body temperature using electronic devices. These devices are fast, safe and some can provide continuous measurements of temperature (Tortora & Grabowski 1996). A selection will now be described in more detail.

Tympanic thermometers

The tympanic membrane shares the same carotid blood supply as the hypothalamus (Klein *et al*. 1993). Measurement of tympanic membrane temperature should therefore reflect core temperature (Woodrow 2000).

The tympanic thermometer (Fig. 10.1), which uses infrared light to detect thermal radiation (Woodrow 2000), is designed for intermittent use, offering a 'one-off' digital reading.

Care should be taken when using the tympanic thermometer as poor technique can render the measurement inaccurate. Temperature differences between the opening of the ear canal and the tympanic membrane can be as much as 2.8°C (Hudak *et al*. 1998). To ensure the temperature measurements are accurate, the tympanic thermometer probe should be positioned to fit snugly in the ear canal. This will prevent ambient air at the opening of the ear canal from entering it, resulting in a false low temperature measurement (Jevon & Jevon 2001).

Although cerumen or earwax can lower measurements by

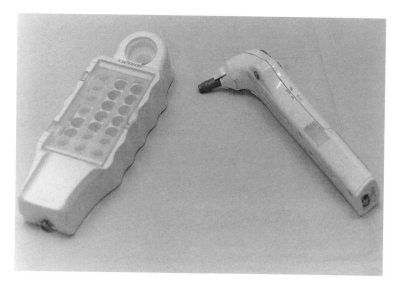

Fig. 10.1 Tympanic thermometer

0.3°C (Doezema *et al*. 1995), it is unlikely that this will affect the management of the patient.

Best practice – tympanic temperature monitoring

Use the same ear for consecutive measurements

Instal a new disposable probe cover for each measurement

Ensure thermometer probe is positioned snugly in the external auditory meatus

Aim the thermometer towards the tympanic membrane

Measure the patient's temperature following manufacturer's instructions

Consider the temperature reading alongside other systemic observations and overall condition of the patient

Store the thermometer following manufacturer's instructions

Jevon & Jevon 2001

Chemical dot thermometers

Chemical dot thermometers are flexible polystyrene strips with a temperature sensor at one end, designed for single oral/axilla use. However their accuracy has been questioned (Erickson *et al*. 1996). These thermometers are unsuitable in patients with hypothermia because their temperature range is restricted to 35.5–40.4°C (O'Toole 1997).

If the oral route is used, the strip should be placed in the sublingual pocket of tissue at the base of the tongue, which is close to the thermoreceptors which rapidly respond to changes in core temperature (Marinin & Wheeler 1997). It is important to ensure that the strip is placed in the sublingual pocket and not in the area under the front of the tongue because there may be a difference in temperature of up to 1.7°C between the two areas (Mallett & Dougherty 2000).

Oral temperature measurements can be affected by the temperature of ingested foods and fluids and by the muscular activity of chewing (Mallett & Dougherty 2000). In addition a respiratory rate of >18 breaths per minute will reduce core temperature values (Marieb 1998).

The axilla is an alternative route for temperature monitoring if the oral route is unsuitable, e.g. in a convulsive patient. However it can be difficult to obtain an accurate and reliable measurement because the site is not close to a major blood vessel and the surface temperature of the skin can be affected by the environment (Woollens 1996).

If the axilla is used, the strip should be placed in the centre of the armpit with the patient's arm positioned firmly against the side of the chest. As the temperature can vary between arms, the same site should be used for serial measurements (Howell 1972).

Regardless of what site is used for temperature measurements, the same one should be consistently used, because switching between different sites can produce measurements that are both misleading and difficult to interpret (Mallett & Dougherty 2000).

Oesophageal/nasopharangeal probes

The oesophageal probe should be accurately positioned in the lower quarter of the oesophagus (Aun 1997). The nasopharangeal temperature can be affected by air leaking around the tracheal tube. Both probes can be interfaced with the patient monitoring system, thus offering an accurate and continuous reading.

Bladder probe

Bladder and pulmonary artery temperature correlate well (Bartlett 1996) and because most critically ill patients require a urinary catheter, this method of measuring body temperature avoids additional invasive equipment.

A thermocouple attached to the distal end of the catheter can interface with the patient monitoring system and offer continuous temperature measurements.

This method of temperature measurement is presumably unreliable if oliguria is present (Woodrow 2000).

Pulmonary artery catheter

Although the pulmonary artery is the gold standard for temperature measurement (Fulbrook 1993), it is highly invasive and its sole use for temperature measurements can not be justified. However if one is inserted, the thermistor sited in the distal end can interface with the patient's monitoring system and can provide continuous temperature measurements.

PHYSIOLOGICAL EFFECTS OF HYPOTHERMIA

Hypothermia, defined as a core temperature of $<35\,^\circ C$ (Chan *et al.* 1998), can occur when the body loses too much heat or cannot maintain its normothermic state. There are a number of risk factors (Table 10.1). Table 10.2 shows the various signs and symptoms of hypothermia at different levels of temperature

Sometimes hypothermia is intentionally induced, e.g. during some cardiac surgery, either by heat exchange through a

Table 10.1 Risk factors for hypothermia

Children
Elderly people
Poor accommodation
Malnourishment
Exposure to a cold environment
Burns
Overdose of medications that lead to coma and immobility
Medications, e.g. benzodiazepines, morphine, barbiturates and vasodilators
Underlying illness, e.g. hypothyroidism
Alcohol abuse
Surgery

Adapted from Kelly *et al.* 2001

heart/lung machine or by surface cooling using ice. The aim is to reduce oxygen and metabolic demands, thus protecting the vital organs during low blood flow periods (Foldy & Gorman 1989).

When monitoring a patient with hypothermia it is important to understand the physiological effects it has on the various systems in the body. The main effects of hypothermia on the bodily systems include:

Cardiovascular system
Initially there is sympathetic stimulation which increases heart rate, BP and cardiac output. However with increasing hypothermia there is progressive cardiovascular depression leading to a reduction in tissue perfusion and oxygenation (Oh 1997) and cardiac arrhythmias, e.g. bradycardia, atrial fibrillation and ventricular fibrillation can become a problem (Resuscitation Council UK 2000). Rough movement and activity should be avoided as this can precipitate a cardiopulmonary arrest. Sometimes the patient's pulse may be difficult to detect.

Table **10**.2 Signs and symptoms of hypothermia at different levels of temperature

37.6°C	'Normal' rectal temperature
37°C	'Normal' oral temperature
36°C	Increased metabolic rate to attempt to balance heat loss
35°C	Shivering maximum at this temperature; hyper-reflexia, dysarthria, delayed cerebration
35°C	Patients usually responsive and with normal blood pressure; lower limit compatible with continued exercise
33–31°C	Retrograde amnesia, consciousness clouded, blood pressure difficult to obtain, pupils dilated, most shivering ceases
30–28°C	Progressive loss of consciousness, increased muscular rigidity, slow pulse and respiration, cardiac arrhythmias develop if heart irritated
27°C	Voluntary motion lost along with pupillary light reflex, deep tendon and skin reflexes; appears dead
26°C	Victims seldom conscious
25°C	Ventricular fibrillation may appear spontaneously
24–21°C	Pulmonary oedema develops (100% mortality in shipwreck victims in World War II)
20°C	Heart standstill
18°C	Lowest adult accidental hypothermic patient with recovery
17°C	Isoelectric EEG
15.2°C	Lowest infant accidental hypothermic patient with recovery
9°C	Lowest artificially cooled hypothermic patient with recovery
4°C	Monkeys revived successfully
1–7°C	Rats and hamsters revived successfully

Reproduced by kind permission of Cambridge University Press from Skinner *et al.* 1997

Respiratory system

Following an initial reflex stimulation of respiration, there is a progressive decrease in respiratory rate, tidal volume and minute volume (Chan *et al*. 1998; Oh 1997) leading to hypoxaemia and hypoxia. Sometimes the patient's respirations may be difficult to detect (Resuscitation Council UK 2000).

Neurological system

Cerebral blood flow reduces at a rate of 7% for each drop in °C (Hudak *et al*. 1998) resulting in confusion, decreased reflexes, cranial nerve deficits and lack of voluntary motion. Increased blood viscosity, decreased oxygen availability, lack of shivering and muscle rigidity also develop (Kelly *et al*. 2001).

Renal system

In mild hypothermia (32°C–35°C) sympathetic activity leads to an increase in cardiac output resulting in a 'cold' diuresis. However with progressive hypothermia, renal blood flow and glomerular filtrate fall. Sodium and water losses may be evident due to metabolic failure of renal tubules (Murphy 1998).

Gastrointestinal system

If the temperature is <34°C, gut motility decreases which can lead to vomiting and malabsorption.

Metabolic system

Metabolic acidosis occurs due to accumulation of lactate and failure to secrete hydrogen ions. Hyperkalaemia resulting from the failure of membrane sodium/potassium pumps and hypoxic liver damage may also occur (Jackson 1998).

Endocrine system

Insulin secretion falls resulting in a failure of glucose utilisation and hyperglycaemia. If hypothermia is prolonged, glycogen stores can become depleted causing hypoglycaemia (Aun 1997).

Haematology

Potential complications include thrombocytopaenia, coagulopathy and disseminated intravascular coagulation (Jackson 1998); splenic sequestration (breaking down or destruction) may also occur, resulting in a decrease in white cell and platelet formation (Aun 1997).

MONITORING PRIORITIES OF A PATIENT WITH HYPOTHERMIA

The monitoring priorities of a patient with hypothermia include:

- regular assessment of vital signs: airway, respirations, blood pressure, pulse and core temperature;
- arterial blood gas analysis;
- ECG monitoring: to detect cardiac arrhythmias;
- urine output measurements;
- blood sugar measurements to detect hypoglycaemia;
- neurological function observations.

Monitoring during rewarming is also important. A patient warmer (Fig. 10.2) is commonly used for rewarming, though other methods are available (Kelly *et al*. 2001). Rewarming should not exceed increases of 0.3–1.2°C per hour in cases of mild hypothermia; but rapid re-warming of >3°C per hour may be necessary if there is severe hypothermia and cardiovascular instability (Carson 1999).

Peripheral vasodilation may complicate active rewarming methods. This could induce hypotension and a further drop in core temperature, the latter increasing the risk of arrhythmias (Murphy 1998). 'Careful monitoring and supportive therapy during rewarming are mandatory' (Aun 1997).

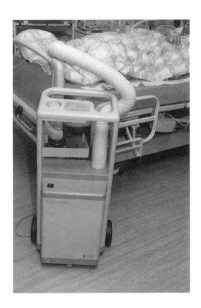

Fig. 10.2 Patient warmer

PHYSIOLOGICAL EFFECTS OF HYPERTHERMIA

Sudden rises in temperature are often caused by infection. However, there are a number of other causes of hyperthermia including:

- hyperthyroidism;
- malignancy;
- drug allergy;
- damage to the central nervous system;
- allergic reaction to blood transfusion;
- heat stroke.

Mallett & Dougherty 2000

Pyrexia in response to infection is a protective mechanism. It inhibits bacterial and viral growth (Ganong 1995), promotes immunity and phagocytosis (Rowsey 1997) and through hypermetabolism promotes tissue repair (Woodrow 2000). Mild pyrexia is generally not treated.

However pyrexia and hypermetabolism can cause physiological stress (Woodrow 2000), e.g. a 13% increase in oxygen consumption with each 1° rise in temperature (Nowak & Handford 1999), a rise in intracranial pressure (Morgan 1990) and cerebral damage (Closs 1992).

Severe hyperthermia or heat stroke is a temperature of >40°C (Aun 1997). It can be caused by MDMA ('ecstasy') (MacConnachie 1997), exposure to a high ambient temperature, vigorous activity and certain drugs (malignant hyperthermia). The main effects of severe hyperthermia on the bodily systems include:

- *neurological system*: confusion, aggression, convulsions and possibly coma;
- *cardiovascular system*: tachycardia and an increase in cardiac output; sometimes hypotension;
- *respiratory system*: tachypnoea and hypoxaemia;
- *renal system*: may precipitate acute renal failure, excessive sweating causes dehydration and oliguria – fluid balance must be monitored;
- *hepatic system*: may precipitate acute liver failure;
- *endocrine system*: may precipitate hypoglycaemia.

Aun 1997

MONITORING PRIORITIES OF A PATIENT WITH HYPERTHERMIA

Monitoring priorities of a patient with hyperthermia include:

- *regular assessment of vital signs*: airway, respirations, blood pressure, pulse and core temperature;
- *arterial blood gas analysis*: particularly important if the patient has malignant hyperthermia as acidosis is common;
- *ECG monitoring*: to detect arrhythmias;
- *urine output* measurements and strict fluid balance;

- *blood sugar* measurements;
- *neurological function* observations.

In addition it is important to monitor any methods used to cool the patient. Core and skin temperature should be closely monitored to avoid overshoot hypothermia and rebound hyperthermia (Aun 1997).

Scenario

A 65-year-old lady was admitted with bronchopneumonia. She looked flushed and was hot to the touch. Her vital signs were BP 130/80, pulse 115, resps 25, tympanic temperature 34.4°C. The tympanic temperature reading is undoubtedly incorrect. What would you do?

There is probably an error with the equipment or technique. The lens on the thermometer was cleaned with a dry wipe. In addition, the end of the probe was placed in the external auditory meatus ensuring a snug fit. The tympanic temperature now showed 38.7°C which was more in line with the patient's clinical condition.

CONCLUSION

A critically ill patient can experience wide fluctuations in body temperature. Severe hypothermia and hyperthermia can be life-threatening. Close monitoring of temperature in the critically ill patient is therefore paramount. It is also paramount to understand the principles of monitoring a hypothermic and hyperthermic patient, particularly during rewarming or cooling procedures.

REFERENCES

Angerami, E. (1980) Epidemiological study of body temperature in patients in a teaching hospital. *International Journal of Nursing Studies* **17**, 91–99.

Aun, C. (1997) Thermal disorders. In: T. Oh, ed. *Intensive Care Manual*, 4th edn. Butterworth Heinemann, Oxford.

Bartlett, E. (1996) Temperature measurement: why and how in intensive care. *Intensive and Critical Care Nursing* **12** (1), 50–54.

Brown, S. (1990) Temperature taking – getting it right. *Nursing Standard* **5** (12), 4–5.

Carson, B. (1999) Successful resuscitation of a 44 year old man with hypothermia. *Journal of Emergency Nursing* **25** (5), 356–360.

Chan, E., Winston, B., Terada, L. & Parsons, P. (1998) *Bedside Critical Care Manual*. Hanley and Belfus, Philadelphia.

Closs, S. (1992) Patients' night-time pain, analgesia provision and sleep after surgery. *International Journal of Nursing Studies* **29** (4), 381–392.

Control of Substances Hazardous to Health Regulations (1999) The Stationery Office, London.

Doezema, D., Lunt, M. & Tandberg, D. (1995) Cerumen occlusion lowers infrared tympanic membrane temperature measurement. *Emergency Medicine* **2** (1), 17–19.

Erickson, R., Meyer, L. & Woo, T. (1996) Accuracy of chemical dot thermometers in critically ill adults and young children. *Image – Journal of Nurse Scholarships* **28** (1), 23–28.

Foldy, S. & Gorman, J. (1989) Perioperative nursing care for congenital cardiac defects. *Critical Care Nursing Clinics of North America* **1**, 289–295.

Fulbrook, P. (1993) Core temperature measurement: a comparison of rectal, axillary and pulmonary artery temperature. *Intensive and Critical Care Nursing* **9** (4), 217–225.

Ganong, W. (1995) *Review of Medical Physiology*, 17th edn. Prentice Hall, London.

Holtzclaw, B. (1992) The febrile response in critical care: state of the science. *Heart and Lung* **21** (5), 482–501.

Howell, T. (1972) Axillary temperature in aged women. *Age and Ageing* **1**, 250–254.

Hudak, C.M., Gallo, B.M. & Morton, P.G. (1998) *Critical Care Nursing: a Holistic Approach*, 7th edn. Lippincott, New York.

Jackson, R. (1998) Physicial Injury In: P. Murphy, ed. *Handbook of Critical Care*. Science Press, London.

Jevon, P. & Jevon, M. (2001) Using a tympanic thermometer. *Nursing Times* **97** (9), 43–44.

Kelly, M., Ewens, B. & Jevon, P. (2001) Hypothermia management. *Nursing Times* **97** (9), 36–37.

Klein, D., Mitchell, C., Petrina, A. *et al.* (1993) A comparison of pulmonary artery, rectal and tympanic membrane temperature measurement in the ICU. *Heart and Lung* **22** (5), 435–441.

MacConnachie, A. (1997) Ecstasy poisoning. *Intensive and Critical Care Nursing* **13** (6), 365–366.

Mallett, J. & Dougherty, L. (2000) eds *The Royal Marsden Hospital Manual of Clinical Nursing Procedures*. Blackwell Science, Oxford.

Marieb, E. (1998) *Human Anatomy and Physiology*, 4th edn. Benjamin Cummings, California.

Marinin, J. & Wheeler, A. (1997) *Medical Care Medicine*, 2nd edn. Williams & Wilkins, London.

Minor, D. & Waterhouse, J. (1981) *Circadian Rhythms and the Human*. Wright, Bristol.

Morgan, S. (1990) A comparison of three methods of managing fever in the neurological patient. *Journal of Neuroscience Nursing* **22** (1), 19–24.

Murphy, P., ed. (1998) *Handbook of Critical Care*. Science Press, London.

Nowak, T. & Handford, A. (1999) *Essentials of Pathophysiology*. McGraw Hill, New York.

Oh, T. ed. (1997) *Intensive Care Manual*, 4th edn. Butterworth Heinemann, Oxford.

O'Toole, S. (1997) Alternatives to mercury thermometers. *Professional Nurse* **12** (11), 783–786.

Resuscitation Council UK (2000) *Advanced Life Support Manual* 4th edn. Resuscitation Council UK, London.

Rowsey, P. (1997) Pathophysiology of fever. Part 2: Relooking at cooling interventions. *Dimensions of Critical Care Nursing* **15** (5), 251–256.

Schmitz, T., Blair, N., Falk, M. *et al.* (1994) A comparison of five methods of temperature measurement in febrile intensive care patients. *American Journal of Intensive Care* **4** (4), 286–292.

Skinner, D.V., Swain, A., Robertson, C. & Rodney Peyton, J.W. (1997) *Cambridge Textbook of Accident and Emergency Medicine*. Cambridge University Press.

Tappen, R. & Andre, S. (1996) Inadvertent hypothermia in elderly surgical patients. *AORN Journal* **63** (3), 639–644.

Tortora, G. & Grabowski, S. (1996) *Principles of Anatomy and Physiology*, 8th edn. Harper Collins, Boston.

Woodrow, P. (2000) *Intensive Care Nursing: A Framework for Practice*. Routledge, London.

Woollens, S. (1996) Temperature measurement devices. *Professional Nurse* **11** (8), 541–547.

Monitoring During Transport

11

INTRODUCTION

It is estimated that over 11 000 critically ill patients require interhospital transport each year (Mackenzie *et al.* 1997 and Intensive Care Society 1997). This number is rising due to the increasing tendency to concentrate such specialist services as trauma, neurosurgery, plastic surgery, cardiothoracics and nephrology in regional centres and the increasing number of transfers for non-clinical reasons.

Despite the large numbers of interhospital transfers, the provision of equipment still remains poor and potentially serious complications frequently occur (Intensive Care Society 1997 and Bion *et al.* 1988). The quality and outcome of the transfer depends on the experience of the transfer team, meticulous clinical preparation and adequate monitoring facilities (Tan 1997). This same level of supervision and preparation is also required for intrahospital transfer of critically ill patients (Intensive Care Society 1997). *Transport of the Critically Ill Adult Patient*, published by the Intensive Care Society (1997), makes recommendations for the organisation and clinical provision of transfers.

The aim of this chapter is to understand the principles of monitoring a critically ill patient during transport.

LEARNING OBJECTIVES

At the end of the chapter the reader will be able to:

❏ list the possible *reasons* for transporting a critically ill patient, both within a hospital and from one hospital to another;

❏ discuss the potential *problems* and *hazards* associated with transport;
❏ discuss what *monitoring equipment* is required for transport;
❏ discuss *what should be monitored* during transport.

REASONS FOR TRANSPORT

Possible reasons for *intrahospital* transport of critically ill patients include:

• diagnostic and therapeutic procedures that can not be undertaken at the bedside, e.g. CT scan;
• need for surgery;
• transfer to ITU/HDU/CCU.

Possible reasons for *interhospital* transport of critically ill patients include:

• non-clinical need, e.g. lack of an ITU bed;
• requirement for specialist services, e.g. renal dialysis;
• requirement for specialist investigations, e.g. angiography;
• requirement for specialist surgery, e.g. neurosurgery, cardiac surgery;
• complex organ support;
• social reasons, e.g. transfer to a hospital nearer to the patient's home.

POTENTIAL PROBLEMS AND HAZARDS ASSOCIATED WITH TRANSPORT

Mortality rates during transport are remarkably low (<1%) (Hinds & Watson 1996). However is still potentially hazardous to transport a critically ill patient, particularly if intensive haemodynamic and respiratory support is required or if it is undertaken by unqualified or inexperienced staff (Bion *et al.* 1988).

The transport of critically ill patients can result in physiological deterioration (Gentleman & Jennett 1981 and Waddell *et al.* 1975). The patient may be unable to tolerate lifting, tipping, abrupt movements, vibration and acceleration/deceleration (Lawler 2000). Accelerational forces and vertical movements can cause cardiovascular instability, particularly in patients who are hypovolaemic or vasodilated due to sepsis, drugs or sedation (Hinds & Watson 1996).

Significant changes in intracranial pressure can be induced by transport, e.g. placing a patient in the head down position when loading onto the ambulance can exacerbate intracranial hypertension (Hinds & Watson 1996). Helicopter transfer may be less hazardous to a critically ill patient, particularly if flown feet first as this will result in a slightly head-up position during acceleration and a slightly head-down position during deceleration. This may minimise the changes in cardiovascular function and intracranial pressure often associated with transport (Kee *et al*. 1992).

An ambulance is probably the worst environment to care for a critically ill patient (Figs 11.1 and 11.2). Space limitations,

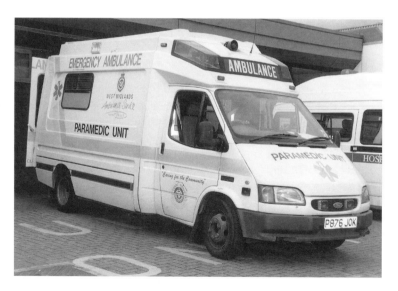

Fig. 11.1 Paramedic ambulance: the most common means of land transport

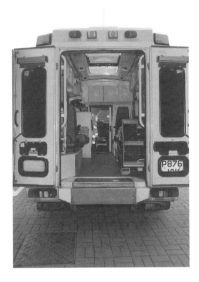

Fig. 11.2 Inside a paramedic ambulance

movement, noise, power sources and lighting can all impose restrictions. Movement of the vehicle can make the performance of even the most routine medical and nursing procedures difficult. A particularly common problem is motion sickness, both for the patient and the staff.

Noise and daylight may render monitors and their alarms unreadable and inaudible. Ambulances rely on battery sources for electrical power. Consequently hospital based equipment which needs alternating current (a.c.) can only be used with its own power source or an a.c./d.c. converter.

Untoward occurrences, including accidental extubation, battery failure, loss of intravenous access and abrupt cessation of vasoactive or sedative agents, are not uncommon. In fact approximately 11–34% of all transports experience equipment problems and mishaps (Carson & Drew 1994; Evans & Winslow 1995; and Smith *et al*. 1990).

Hazards associated with air transport

The hazards encountered with air transport are dependent to a degree on the mode of transport (helicopter or aeroplane) and can be summarised as follows.

- *Expansion of gas in closed cavities*: as atmospheric pressure falls with increasing altitude, the volume occupied by gas rises; clinically this will result in trapped gases expanding. This will exacerbate a pneumothorax. In addition air in a tracheal tube cuff is susceptible to these changes; either gently fill the cuff with normal saline or continuously monitor the cuff pressure during altitude changes.
- *Fluid loss*: a fall in atmospheric pressure can cause fluid to extravasate from the intravascular to the interstitial space resulting in oedema, hypotension and tachycardia; further, the effects of dehydration can be exacerbated (Hinds & Watson 1996).
- *Hypoxia*: increasing altitude causes a fall in the partial pressure of oxygen which can lead to a fall in alveolar oxygen and hypoxia.
- *Temperature control*: heating in helicopters can be particularly difficult. In addition the patient may be exposed to the environment when being transferred to and from the aircraft.
- *Noise*: will cause sensory deprivation; in particular helicopter noise can interfere with monitoring, especially audible warning devices (Kee *et al*. 1992).
- *Vibration*: can make monitoring difficult and can cause problems with gravity dependent intravenous fluid administration.
- *Visibility*: may be reduced; this together with the noise can make monitoring even more difficult; visual alarms may be obscured.
- *Unfamiliar environment*: can be stressful for staff.

PATIENT MONITORING EQUIPMENT REQUIRED FOR TRANSPORT

Determining what monitoring equipment should be taken will depend on the condition of the patient and the available resources on the mode of transport. Any equipment taken should be:

- lightweight, yet durable and robust;
- restrained, yet easily accessible;
- regularly checked (Gilligan 1997);
- battery powered if electrical (with battery life display).

Ideally equipment should have both audible and visual alarms. A small versatile portable monitor such as a Propaq (Fig. 11.3) is invaluable. Depending on what is required, recordings of ECG, oxygen saturation, non-invasive blood pressure, temperature, invasive pressures and capnography

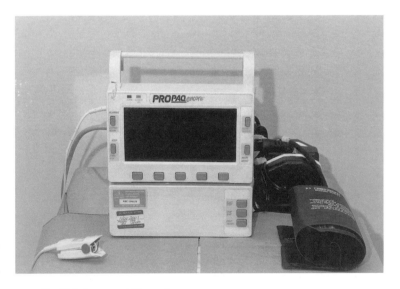

Fig. 11.3 Propaq portable monitor

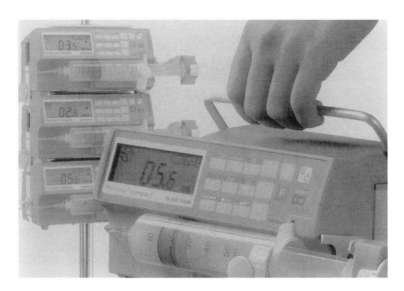

Fig. 11.4 Infusion pumps

can be taken. Capnography is recommended as a mandatory requirement by the Intensive Care Society (1997).

Infusion pumps (Fig. 11.4) and appropriate medications should be available. In particular it is important to ensure that essential infusions, e.g. vasoactive drugs do not run out during transfer. Although a mobile phone should ideally be available to help with communications, any possible effect on monitoring equipment should be checked. If air transport is being undertaken, *always* check with the pilot before using a mobile phone, as mobiles can interfere with aircraft navigation and avionics.

MONITORING DURING TRANSFER

The standard of care and monitoring during transport, which will depend on the individual needs of the patient, should be maintained at the same level as on the Intensive Care Unit.

The Intensive Care Society (1997) makes the following recommendations.

- *Arterial oxygenation, ECG, and arterial pressure* should be monitored in every patient.
- *Invasive arterial monitoring* is preferable to non-invasive as the latter is sensitive to motion.
- *Central venous pressure, pulmonary artery wedge pressure or intracranial pressure* may be required in some patients; interpretation may however, be difficult in a moving ambulance and treatment is therefore difficult to control.
- If the patient is being *mechanically ventilated* the oxygen supply and airway pressure should be monitored; a means for detecting disconnection should be established (one third of hospitals do not have a ventilator disconnector alarm) (Knowles *et al.* 1999).
- *End tidal CO_2 measurement* is desirable particularly in patients with cerebral injury regardless of the cause, though fewer than 50% of hospitals have the facility to undertake this during transport (Knowles *et al.* 1999).
- *Temperature* should be monitored if it is abnormal, during long journeys or in cold weather.

Assessment of adequacy of ventilation is notoriously inaccurate in an ambulance (Knowles *et al.* 1999). There are now sophisticated portable ventilators which can maintain the most dependent patient, without compromising their respiratory rate, for limited periods of time (Fig. 11.5). These offer different modes and run on a battery, requiring only an oxygen cylinder source.

If parenteral nutrition is halted it is recommended to administer 10% glucose to avoid rebound hypoglycaemia (Gilligan 1997). The blood glucose should be closely monitored during transfer.

As well as monitoring the patient, it is also important to monitor the equipment continuously, particularly alarms. Intravenous infusions should also be closely monitored to

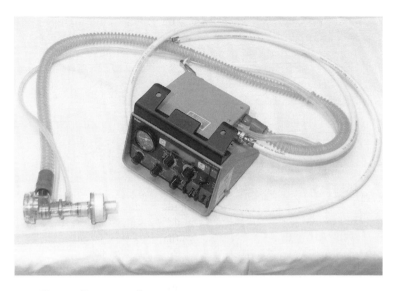

Fig. 11.5 Transport ventilator

ensure that the prescribed dose is being administered and that they have not run out.

Unskilled or inexperienced staff may not recognise or rectify problems (Braman *et al.* 1987). Experienced staff should be in attendance, e.g. a senior ICU nurse and an anaesthetist, who should have the necessary skills to manage any sudden and unexpected outcome.

CONCLUSION

Transporting a critically ill patient can be fraught with difficulties and is potentially hazardous. Therefore it is important to justify any transport whether it is intrahospital or interhospital. Knowledge of potential problems and hazards associated with transport is essential if patient monitoring during transport is to be undertaken accurately and effectively, thus minimising morbidity and mortality.

Risks are reduced when there is meticulous clinical preparation, appropriate equipment available for use and when transfer is undertaken by experienced staff familiar with the transfer environment. The same level of supervision and preparation is also important when critically ill patients are transferred between departments within a hospital.

ACKNOWLEDGEMENT

Some text in this chapter has been reproduced, with kind permission, from Jevon, P. & Ewens, B. (2001) Care of patients on the move. *Nursing Times* **97** (4), 35–6.

REFERENCES

Bion, J.F., Wilson, I.H. & Taylor, P.A. (1988) Transporting critically ill patients by ambulance: audit by sickness scoring. *British Medical Journal* **296**, 170–174.

Braman, S., Dunn, S., Amico, C.A. & Millman, R.P. (1987) Complications of intrahospital transport in critically ill patients. *Annals of Internal Medicine* **107**, 469–473.

Carson, B. (1999) Successful resuscitation of a 44 year old man with hypothermia. *Journal of Emergency Nursing* **25** (5), 356–360.

Carson, K.J. & Drew, B.J. (1994) Electrocardiographic changes in critically ill adults during intrahospital transport. *Progress in Cardiovascular Nursing* **9** (4), 4–12.

Evans, A. & Winslow, E.H. (1995) Oxygen saturation and hemo-dynamic response in critically ill, mechanically ventilated adults during intrahospital transport. *American Journal of Critical Care* **4** (2), 106–111.

Gentleman, D. & Jennett, B. (1981) Hazards of inter-hospital transfer of comatose head-injured patients. *The Lancet* **1**, 853–855.

Gilligan, J. (1997) Transport of the critically ill. In: T. Oh ed., *Intensive Care Manual* 4th edn. Butterworth-Heinemann, Oxford.

Hinds, C.J. & Watson, D. (1996) *Intensive Care, A Concise Textbook*, 2nd edn. W.B. Saunders, London.

Intensive Care Society (1997) *Guidelines for the Transport of Critically Ill Patients*. Intensive Care Society, London.

Kee, S.S., Ramage, C.M.H., Mednel, P. & Bristow, A.S.E. (1992) Interhospital transfers by helicopter: the first 50 patients of the Carelight project. *Journal of the Royal Society of Medicine* **85**, 29–31.

Knowles, P.R., Bryden, P.C., Kishen, R. & Gwinnutt, C.L. (1999)

Meeting the standards for interhospital transfer of adults with severe head injury in the United Kingdom. *Anaesthesia* **54** (3), 283–288.

Lawler, P.G. (2000) Transfer of critically ill patients: Part 1 – Physiological concepts. *Care of the Critically Ill* **16** (2), 61–65.

Lee, A., Lum, M.E., Beehan, S.J. & Hillman, K.M. (1996) Interhospital transfers: decision making in critical care areas. *Critical Care Medicine* **24** (4), 618–622.

Mackenzie, P.A., Smith, E.A. & Wallace, P.G.M. (1997) Transfer of adults between intensive care units in the United Kingdom: postal survey. *British Medical Journal* **314**, 455–456.

Smith, I., Fleming, S. & Cernaianu, A. (1990) Mishaps during transport from the intensive care unit. *Critical Care Medicine* **18** (2), 278–281.

Tan, T.K. (1997) Interhospital and intrahospital transfer of the critically ill patient. *Singapore Medical Journal* **36** (6), 244–248.

Waddell, G., Scott, P.D.R. & Lees, N.W. (1975) Effects of ambulance transport in critically ill patients. *British Medical Journal* **1**, 386–389.

Record Keeping

INTRODUCTION

An accurate written record detailing all aspects of patient monitoring is important, not only because it forms an integral part of the nursing management of the patient, but also because it can help to protect practitioners if defence of their actions is required. Most of the text in this chapter is based on *Guidelines for Records and Record Keeping* published by the UKCC (1998) (Fig. 12.1).

The aim of this chapter is to understand the principles of good record keeping.

LEARNING OBJECTIVES

At the end of the chapter the reader will be able to:

❏ discuss the importance of good record keeping;
❏ outline the principles of good record keeping;
❏ outline the importance of auditing records;
❏ discuss the legal issues associated with record keeping.

IMPORTANCE OF GOOD RECORD KEEPING

> 'Record keeping is an integral part of nursing, midwifery and health visiting practice. It is a tool of professional practice and one which should help the care process. It is not separate from this process and it is not an optional extra to be fitted in if circumstances allow.'
>
> UKCC 1998

Good record keeping will help to protect the welfare of both the patient and practitioner by promoting:

Guidelines for records and record keeping

United Kingdom Central Council
for Nursing, Midwifery and Health Visiting

Protecting the public through professional standards

Fig. 12.1 *Guidelines for records and record keeping* UKCC (1998)

- high standards of clinical care;
- continuity of care through better communication and dissemination of information between members of the inter-professional healthcare team;
- early detection of problems, such as changes in the patient's condition;
- an accurate account of treatment and care planning and delivery.

The quality of record keeping is also a reflection on the standard of nursing practice: good record keeping is an indication that the practitioner is professional and skilled while poor record keeping often highlights wider problems with the individual's practice (UKCC 1998).

PRINCIPLES OF GOOD RECORD KEEPING

There are a number of factors that underpin good record keeping. The patient's records should:

- be factual, consistent and accurate;
- be updated as soon as possible after any recordable event;
- provide current information on the care and condition of the patient;
- be documented clearly and in such a way that the text can not be erased;
- be consecutive and accurately dated, timed and signed (including a printed signature);
- have any alterations and additions dated, timed and signed; all original entries should be clearly legible;
- not include abbreviations, jargon, meaningless phrases, irrelevant speculation and offensive subjective statements;
- still be legible if photocopied;
- identify any problems identified and most importantly the action taken to rectify them.

It is important to record all aspects of patient monitoring. Some observations will be recorded on the patient's observation charts (e.g. the ICU Observation Chart and the Standard Observation Chart, see Fig. 12.2). Dates and times should be clearly visible and standard coloured ink following local protocols should be used. It is also important to ensure that an accurate record is made in the patient's notes. In particular it is important to include interventions and any response to the interventions.

Best practice – record keeping

Records must be:

factual

legible

clear

concise

accurate

signed

timed

dated

Drew *et al.* 2000

IMPORTANCE OF AUDITING RECORDS

Audit can play an important role in ensuring quality of health care. In particular it can help to improve the process of record keeping. By auditing records the standard can be evaluated and any areas for improvement and staff development identified. Audit tools should be developed at a local level to monitor the standards of record keeping.

Audit should primarily be aimed at serving the interests of the patient rather than the organisation (UKCC 1998). A system of peer review may also be of value. Whatever audit system is used, the confidentiality of patients' information applies to audit just as it does to record keeping.

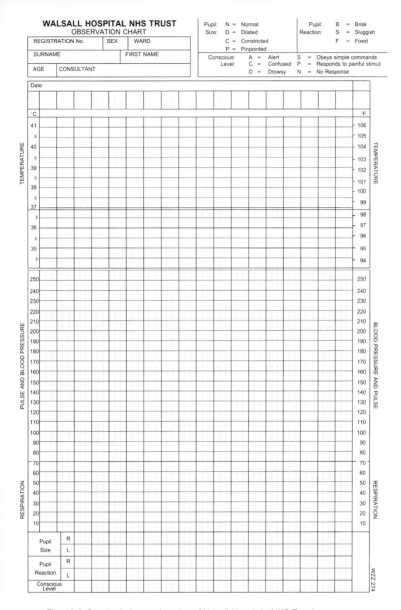

Fig. 12.2 Standard observation chart (Walsall Hospitals NHS Trust)

LEGAL ISSUES ASSOCIATED WITH RECORD KEEPING

The patient's records are occasionally required as evidence before a court of law, by the Health Service Commissioner or in order to investigate a complaint at a local level. Sometimes they may be requested by the UKCC's Professional Conduct Committee when investigating complaints related to misconduct. Care plans, diaries and anything that makes reference to the patient's care may be required as evidence (UKCC 1998).

What constitutes a legal document is often a cause for concern. Any document requested by the court becomes a legal document (Dimond 1994), e.g. nursing records, medical records, X-rays, laboratory reports, observation charts; in fact any document which may be relevant to the case.

If any of the documents are missing, the writer of the records may be cross-examined as to the circumstances of their disappearance (Dimond 1994). 'Medical records are not proof of the truth of the facts stated in them but the maker of the records may be called to give evidence as to the truth as to what is contained in them' (Dimond 1994).

'The approach to record keeping which courts of law adopt tends to be that if it is not recorded, it has not been done' (UKCC 1998). Professional judgement is required when deciding what is relevant and what needs to be recorded, particularly if the patient's clinical condition is apparently unchanging and no record has been made of the care that has been delivered.

A registered nurse has both a professional and a legal duty of care. Consequently when keeping records it is important to be able to demonstrate that:

- a comprehensive nursing assessment of the patient has been undertaken including care that has been planned and provided;
- relevant information is included together with any measures that have been taken in response to changes in the patient's condition;

- the duty of care owed to the patient has been honoured and that no acts or omissions have compromised the patient's safety;
- arrangements have been made for ongoing care of the patient.

The registered nurse is also accountable for any delegation of record keeping to members of the interprofessional team who are not registered practitioners. For example, if record keeping is delegated to a preregistration student nurse or a healthcare assistant, competence to perform the task must be ensured and adequate supervision provided. All such entries must be countersigned.

The Access to Health Records Act 1990 gives patients the right of access to their manually maintained health records which were made after 1 November 1991. The Data Protection Act 1998 gives patients the right to access their computer-held records. Sometimes it is necessary to withhold information, if it could affect the physical or mental well-being of the patient or if it would breach another patient's confidentiality (UKCC 1998). If the decision to withhold information is made, justification for doing so must be clearly recorded in the patient's notes.

CONCLUSION

When monitoring a critically ill patient it is important to ensure good record keeping. Good record keeping is both the product of good teamwork and an important tool in promoting high quality health care.

REFERENCES

Dimond, B. (1994) *Legal Aspects in Midwifery.* Books for Midwives. Midwifery Press, Cheshire.

Drew, D., Jevon, P. & Raby, M. (2000) *Resuscitation of the Newborn.* Butterworth Heinemann, Oxford.

UKCC (1998) *Guidelines for Records and Record Keeping.* UKCC, London.

Index